STUDY GUIDE
for the
ANATOMY *and*
PHYSIOLOGY LEARNING
SYSTEM

Fourth Edition

Edith Applegate, MS
Professor of Science and Mathematics
Kettering College of Medical Arts
Kettering, OH

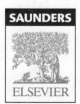

SAUNDERS

ELSEVIER

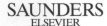

SAUNDERS
ELSEVIER

3251 Riverport Lane
St. Louis, Missouri 63043

STUDY GUIDE FOR THE ANATOMY AND   978-1-4377-0394-8
PHYSIOLOGY LEARNING SYSTEM

Executive Editor: Suzi Epstein
Developmental Editor: Lynda Huenefeld
Publishing Services Manager: Deborah L. Vogel
Senior Project Manager: Ann E. Rogers
Design Direction: Gopal Venkatram

Printed in the United States of America

Last digit is the print number: 12

Note to Students

Dear Student,

I am excited about Anatomy and Physiology. I find the subject fascinating. I also realize that many students become overwhelmed and frustrated because there is so much to learn, so I have prepared this workbook to help you master, and hopefully enjoy, your study of anatomy and physiology. It contains many tools to help you learn.

Each chapter begins with **learning exercises** in a variety of formats. Some are questions to answer or statements to complete. Others are paragraphs in which you will fill in the missing words, matching exercises, and diagrams to label and color. Many of the exercises ask you to write key words because this helps you learn to spell the words correctly. A small set of colored pencils will be useful because many of the labeling exercises suggest that you color code some of the structures on the diagram.

After the exercises there are **review questions** to lead you through the material again. Now you are ready for the **chapter quiz**. You can use this as a measuring tool to see how well you are doing.

To close each chapter in the workbook, I have prepared a word puzzle that relates to the topics in the chapter. These are for those moments when you don't feel like studying and know you should. Maybe the puzzles will get you in the mood. I had a lot of fun preparing the **Fun & Games** pages, and I hope you have fun doing them. My philosophy is that you can learn and have fun at the same time.

Carrying this study guide to and from class may help your cardiovascular system, but it won't help you learn anatomy and physiology unless you actually **use** it. You learn better when you are actively involved, and this study guide provides a means for your participation in your learning process. It offers another method of study after you have studied your notes and textbook. The study guide also provides a focus for small group study with your peers. Use it. You'll be glad you did.

I hope you enjoy your study of the human body. I would like to hear from you and have your comments and suggestions about ways to improve **The Anatomy and Physiology Learning System**. In closing, I offer my best wishes for success in this course, in your selected curriculum, and in your chosen career.

Sincerely,
Edith Applegate
Professor of Science and Mathematics
Kettering College of Medical Arts

Contents

1 Introduction to Anatomy and Physiology

LEARNING EXERCISES

Anatomy and Physiology

1. The study of morphology or structure of organisms is called _____.

2. _____ is the scientific study of body functions.

3. Anatomy and physiology are interrelated because the structure of a body part influences its _____

   and function has an effect on _____.

4. Identify the specialty areas of anatomy and physiology that are described below by writing the name of the specialty area on the line preceding the description.

   A. _____ Study of external features

   B. _____ Study of cellular structure

   C. _____ Study of prenatal development

   D. _____ Study of the body's defense against disease

   E. _____ Study of drug action in the body

   F. _____ Study of structural and functional changes associated with disease

Levels of Organization

1. The six levels of organization in the body, in sequence from the simplest to the most complex, are

   _____, _____, _____, _____,

   _____, _____.

2. The basic living unit of all organisms is the _____.

3. A _____ is a collection of cells with similar structure and function.

1

Organic Systems

Write the name of the organ system that corresponds to each of the descriptions.

Cardiovascular   Muscular   Urinary
Lymphatic   Skeletal   Integumentary
Respiratory   Endocrine   Reproductive
Digestive   Nervous

1. _____ Consists of the skin, hair, and sweat glands

2. _____ Bones and ligaments

3. _____ Processes food into usable molecules

4. _____ Trachea, bronchi, and lungs

5. _____ Removes nitrogenous wastes from the blood

6. _____ Glands that secrete hormones

7. _____ Cleanses lymph and returns it to the blood

8. _____ Brain, spinal cord, nerves, and sense receptors

9. _____ Blood, heart, and blood vessels

10. _____ Part of the body's defense system

11. _____ Esophagus, stomach, liver, and pancreas

12. _____ Transmits impulses to coordinate body activities

13. _____ Chemical messengers that regulate body activities

14. _____ Transports nutrients, hormones, and oxygen

15. _____ Regulates fluid and chemical content of the body

16. _____ Produces movement and maintains posture

17. _____ Tonsils, spleen, lymph nodes, and thymus

18. _____ Protective covering of the body

19. _____ Forms the framework of the body

20. _____ Ovaries and testes

Life Processes

1. List 10 life processes that distinguish living organisms from nonliving forms.

2. _____ is the phase of metabolism in which complex substances are broken down into simpler ones.

3. Define anabolism.

Environmental Requirements for Life

1. List five physical factors from the environment that are essential to human life.

Homeostasis

Write the term that is defined by each of the following phrases.

1. _____ Maintenance of a relatively stable internal environment

2. _____ Any condition that disrupts homeostasis

3. _____ Action that has an effect opposite to a deviation from normal; action to maintain homeostasis

4. _____ Mechanisms that stimulate or amplify changes

Anatomic Terms

1. Describe the anatomic position by stating the position of each of the following parts:

   A. Body is _____

   B. Face is _____

   C. Arms are _____

   D. Palms are _____

   E. Feet and toes are _____

2. Provide the directional term that correctly completes each statement.

   A. The nose is _____ to the mouth.

   B. The elbow is _____ to the wrist.

   C. Muscles are _____ to the skin.

   D. The heart is _____, or in front of, the vertebral column.

   E. The _____ pericardium covers the heart.

3. Name the plane that:

   A. _____ Divides the body into right and left halves.

   B. _____ Divides the body into superior and inferior portions.

   C. _____ Divides the body into anterior and posterior portions.

   D. _____ Divides the body into right and left portions.

4. Name the most specific body cavity that is described by each of the following phrases:

   A. _____ Contains the cranial and spinal cavities.

   B. _____ Contains the thoracic and abdominopelvic cavities.

   C. _____ Contains the brain.

   D. _____ Contains the heart and lungs.

   E. _____ Contains the liver, stomach, and spleen.

   F. _____ Contains the spinal cord.

   G. _____ Contains the urinary bladder and rectum.

LABELING AND COLORING EXERCISES

1. Each of the following squares represents a plane of the body. Color the sagittal plane red, the horizontal (transverse) plane blue, and the frontal (coronal) plane yellow. *R*, Right, *L*, left; *A*, anterior; *P*, posterior; *S*, superior, *I*, inferior.

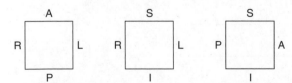

Chapter **1** **Introduction to Anatomy and Physiology**

2. In Figure 1-1, color the dorsal body cavity red and the ventral body cavity blue. Identify the subdivisions of each cavity as indicated.

A. _____

B. _____

C. _____

D. _____

E. _____

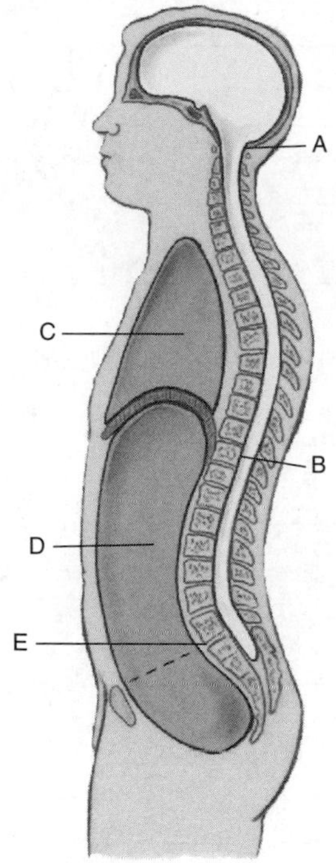

Figure 1-1 Body cavities.

3. Label the nine regions of the abdomen indicated in Figure 1-2.

A. _____

B. _____

C. _____

D. _____

E. _____

F. _____

G. _____

H. _____

I. _____

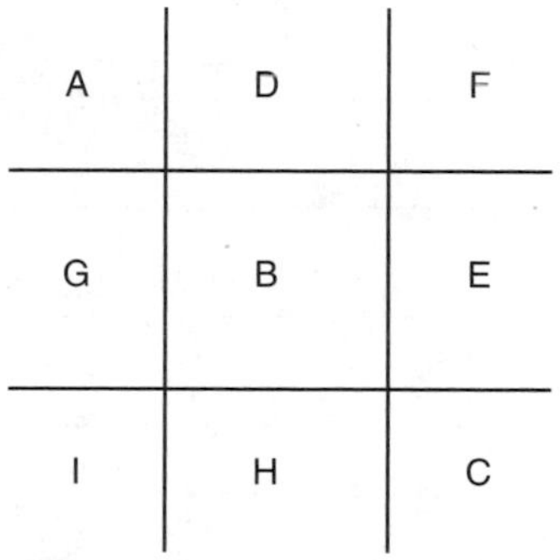

Figure 1-2 Nine abdominal regions.

4. Label the body regions indicated in Figure 1-3 and Figure 1-4.

A. _____

B. _____

C. _____

D. _____

E. _____

F. _____

G. _____

H. _____

I. _____

J. _____

K. _____

L. _____

M. _____

N. _____

O. _____

P. _____

Q. _____

R. _____

S. _____

T. _____

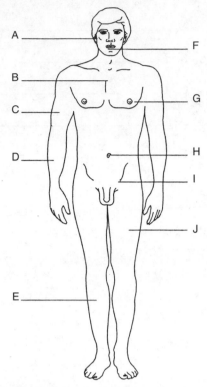

Figure 1-3   Anterior view.

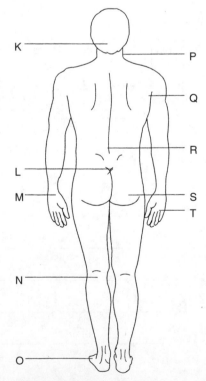

Figure 1-4   Posterior view.

REVIEW QUESTIONS

1. What is the relationship between anatomy and physiology?

2. Starting with the simplest or smallest level, name in sequence the six levels of organization in the human body.

3. List the 11 organ systems in the body, and describe the general functions of each one.

4. What are five characteristics that distinguish living from nonliving forms?

5. What are five characteristics that distinguish advanced life forms, such as humans, from other living forms?

6. Name five environmental factors that are necessary to maintain human life.

7. What is meant by homeostasis, and how is it maintained?

8. How does positive feedback differ from negative feedback?

9. Describe the position of the head, arms, hands, and feet when the body is in anatomic position.

10. Use these directional terms to write sentences that describe the relative positions of the indicated body parts:
    A. Superior/inferior (mouth and nose)

    B. Anterior/posterior (spinal cord and heart)

    C. Medial/lateral (ears and eyes)

Chapter **1** **Introduction to Anatomy and Physiology**

D. Proximal/distal (elbow and wrist)

E. Superficial/deep (skin and muscles)

11. How are you dividing the body when you cut on each of the following planes?

A. Coronal plane

B. Transverse plane

C. Sagittal plane

12. What are the two major body cavities, and which one is larger?

13. What makes up the axial portion of the body?

14. Use two horizontal and two vertical lines to form a grid (like tic-tac-toe), and then identify each of the nine areas of the abdominopelvic region.

15. Use two anatomic terms that pertain to specific regions of the head, the arm, the thorax, the abdomen, and the lower extremity.

16. Using the word parts given in this chapter, write a word that means the process of cutting apart.

VOCABULARY PRACTICE

For each of the following terms, underline the root and write the definition of the root in the space provided.

1. adenitis _____

2. carcinoma _____

3. cephalad _____

4. integument _____

5. visceral _____

6. renal _____

7. pathology _____

8. homeostasis _____

9. proximal _____

10. gastritis _____

8

11. For each of the following terms, circle the prefix and write the definition of the prefix in the space provided.

A. subcutaneous _____   F. macrocephaly _____

B. intracellular _____   G. anteversion _____

C. hypersensitive _____   H. abduct _____

D. anorexia _____   I. intercostal _____

E. epigastric _____   J. pericardium _____

12. For each of the following terms, circle the suffix and write the definition of the suffix in the space provided.

A. cardiac _____   F. anatomist _____

B. physiology _____   G. leukocytosis _____

C. arthralgia _____   H. tracheotomy _____

D. dermatitis _____   I. hyperthyroidism _____

E. electrocardiogram _____   J. colonoscopy _____

13. Match the definitions on the left with the correct clinical term from the column on the right by placing the corresponding letter in the space before the definition.

A. _____ Evidence of disease that can be evaluated or observed by someone other than the patient

B. _____ Nature of a disease or structure that is based on the name of an individual

C. _____ Prediction of the course of a disease and the recovery rate

D. _____ A combination of signs and symptoms occurring together that characterize a disease

E. _____ Evidence of disease that can only be evaluated by the patient

1. Eponym
2. Prognosis
3. Sign
4. Symptom
5. Syndrome

14. Write the meaning of each of the following clinical abbreviations.

A. Abd _____   F. PRN _____

B. H&P _____   G. C _____

C. BP _____   H. tab _____

D. Dx _____   I. mg _____

E. ENT _____   J. ant _____

15. Spelling is important in scientific and medical applications because only one or two incorrect letters can change the meaning. Six of the following words from this chapter are misspelled. Place a check mark (√) in the space before the word if it is spelled correctly. Write the correct spelling in the space if it is spelled incorrectly.

A. homeostasis _____   F. prognosis _____

B. saggital _____   G. limfatic _____

C. endocryn _____   H. visceral _____

D. phyziology _____   I. hypochondriac _____

E. epinime _____   J. addominopelvic _____

16. Using word parts from this chapter, write words that have the following meanings.

A. Pertaining to internal organs _____

B. Process of making a recording of the heart _____

C. Study of the stomach _____

D. Pertaining to the back _____

E. Study of disease _____

TESTING COMPREHENSION

Circle the letter that corresponds with the correct answer.

1. The smallest unit of organization that is *living* is (a) chemical, (b) cell, (c) tissue, (d) organ.

2. Which of the following does *not* represent a correct grouping of organ system/part of system/function? (a) integumentary/skin/cover and protect, (b) endocrine/ductless glands/regulate metabolic activity, (c) respiratory/lungs/exchange of gases, (d) lymphatic/heart/defense against disease.

3. Which of the following correctly lists three physical factors from the environment that are necessary to sustain human life? (a) oxygen, metabolism, respiration; (b) water, organization, excretion; (c) oxygen, water, anabolism; (d) oxygen, water, pressure.

4. Which one of the following does *not* pertain to a negative feedback mechanism? (a) When blood pressure decreases, the heart beats faster to increase blood pressure. (b) When air temperature increases, sweating increases. (c) When blood sugar level decreases, the hunger center in the brain is stimulated. (d) When deviations from normal occur, this mechanism increases the deviations.

5. In anatomic position, (a) your body is erect, arms are behind your back; (b) your eyes are facing the same direction as your palms; (c) you are sitting down with feet forward; (d) feet are forward and palms are in the opposite direction.

6. Which of the following means closer to a point of attachment or origin? (a) superficial, (b) anterior, (c) proximal, (d) medial.

10

Chapter **1** **Introduction to Anatomy and Physiology**

7. The region that is in the midline, superior to the umbilical region, is the (a) hypogastric, (b) hypochondria, (c) lumbar, (d) epigastric.

8. The appendicular portion of the body includes the (a) head and neck, (b) arms and legs, (c) thorax and abdomen, (d) brain and spinal cord.

9. The exchange of oxygen and carbon dioxide between the outside air and the blood would be included in the study of the (a) anatomy of the respiratory system, (b) physiology of the respiratory system, (c) anatomy of the cardiovascular system, (d) physiology of the cardiovascular system.

10. A patient went to the emergency room with pain in the abdominal region. Tests revealed a bleeding ulcer in the stomach. The stomach is a part of the (a) muscular system, (b) cardiovascular system, (c) lymphatic system, (d) digestive system.

11. Jamie sprained his ankle while playing basketball. The fact that he felt pain is called (a) movement; (b) differentiation; (c) responsiveness; (d) metabolism.

12. The two major cavities of the body are the (a) thoracic and abdominal; (b) anterior and posterior; (c) sagittal and coronal; (d) dorsal and ventral.

13. The following is an example of a positive feedback mechanism: (a) maintaining a normal blood pressure; (b) maintaining a constant body temperature; (c) increasing strength of uterine contractions during childbirth; (d) becoming thirsty when the body fluid volume decreases.

14. Jason mowed lawns in the summer to earn money for college. On hot days he perspires a lot and the evaporation of the perspiration helps cool the body. This is an example of (a) metabolism, (b) negative feedback, (c) anabolism, (d) respiration.

15. The lungs are located in the thoracic cavity. What term best describes their relationship to the diaphragm: (a) superior, (b) inferior, (c) lateral, (d) distal.

16. The heart is located in the mediastinum. Which of the following does *not* describe the location of the mediastinum? (a) ventral body cavity, (b) superior to the diaphragm, (c) in the epigastric region, (d) thoracic cavity.

17. Tammy fell when riding her bicycle and fractured a bone in the carpal region. Where is this region? (a) arm, (b) leg, (c) ankle, (d) wrist.

18. The portion of the brachial region that is closer to the elbow than the axillary region is the (a) superficial region, (b) proximal region, (c) distal region, (d) superior region.

19. Which body regions are inferior to the costal region? (a) sternal and otic, (b) inguinal and pelvic, (c) cervical and occipital, (d) mammary and buccal.

20. The region behind the knee is the (a) patellar region, (b) antecubital region, (c) crural region, (d) popliteal region.

21. A visual examination of the stomach is (a) gastritis, (b) gastroscopy, (c) gastroenteritis, (d) gastralgia.

22. The study of disease is called (a) pathology, (b) physiology, (c) histology, (d) immunology.

23. The suffix -*algia* means (a) the study of, (b) pain, (c) inflammation, (d) process or condition.

24. Dr. Joe Stanley informed Linda that her prognosis was excellent. What did he mean? (a) She had a disappearance of symptoms without achieving a cure. (b) Her disease had a sudden onset, severe symptoms, and short duration. (c) There was a good chance of recovery. (d) The disease would continue over a long period of time with little change in symptoms.

25. Susan was diagnosed as having an adenocarcinoma. This means that she had (a) a cancerous tumor of a gland, (b) inflammation of a gland, (c) an abnormal secretion from a gland, (d) a benign cyst on a gland.

A STEP BEYOND

Go a step beyond the ordinary and learn more about a topic that is related to this chapter but not discussed in detail in the textbook. Select one of the following topics, or one suggested by your instructor, and write a brief paper (250 words minimum), create a poster, or develop a short presentation (approximately 4 to 5 minutes) that focuses on your selection. Suggested topics for this chapter include the following:

1. *History of anatomy.* Investigate the history of anatomy from the fifth century to the second century BCE. The history should include contributions by Hippocrates, Aristotle, Herophilus, Erasistratus, Alcmaeon, and Empedocles.

2. *Positive feedback.* Describe two examples of positive feedback loops in human physiology.

FUN & GAMES

Word Scramble

Determine the word that fits each definition, and then write the word in the spaces below the definition, one letter per space. The letters in the boxes form a scrambled word. Unscramble the letters to create a word that matches the final definition in each section.

1. Plane that divides the body into right and left portions

2. Constant internal environment

3. Study of structure

4. Inferior cavity of the dorsal body cavity

5. Plane that divides the body into anterior and posterior portions

Letters to use for final word: _____

Final definition: Abdominal region superior to the umbilical region

_____

6. A word formed from the initial letters of the successive parts of a compound term

7. Name of a disease, structure, or procedure that is based on the name of an individual

8. Identification of a disease

9. Partial or complete disappearance of the symptoms of a disease without achieving a cure

Letters to use for final word: _____

Final definition: A combination of signs and symptoms occurring together that characterize a specific disease.

_____

2 Chemistry, Matter, and Life

LEARNING EXERCISES

Elements

1. Matter is defined as _____

_____

2. An element is defined as _____

_____

3. Write the chemical symbol for each of the following elements.

_____ Hydrogen   _____ Magnesium   _____ Carbon

_____ Oxygen   _____ Potassium   _____ Phosphorus

4. Identify the element that is represented by each of the following symbols.

_____ Na   _____ N

_____ Ca   _____ Fe

_____ Cl   _____ S

Structure of Atoms

1. Draw a simple diagram that illustrates the structure of an oxygen atom, which has an atomic number = 8 and a mass number = 16.

2. Fill in the information that is missing from the following table.

Particle	Location	Charge	Mass
		0	
			Negligible
Proton			

3. How many protons, neutrons, and electrons are in an atom of potassium, which has an atomic number = 19 and a mass number = 39?

_____ Protons   _____ Neutrons   _____ Electrons

4. The most stable atoms have _____ electrons in their highest energy level.

Isotopes

1. Atoms of a given element that have different atomic weights are called _____. The difference in atomic weight is due to a difference in the number of _____.

2. Unstable isotopes that emit atomic radiation are called _____.

Chemical Bonds

Match each of the following terms with the correct definition below.

1. _____   Intermolecular bond

2. _____   Ion with a negative charge

3. _____   Ion with a positive charge

4. _____   Bond between anions and cations

5. _____   Bond in which electrons are shared

6. _____   Bond between polar covalent molecules

A. ionic bond

B. covalent bond

C. hydrogen bond

D. anion

E. cation

Compounds and Molecules

Indicate whether each of the following refers to an atom, a molecule, or a compound.

1. _____   Smallest unit of an element that retains the properties of that element

2. _____   Formed when two or more atoms are held together by chemical bonds

3. _____   Formed when two or more different atoms are chemically combined in a definite ratio

4. _____   Smallest unit of a compound that retains the properties of that compound

5. The molecular formula for calcium carbonate, one of the mineral salts in bone, is $CaCO_3$. Name the elements in this compound, and tell how many atoms of each element are present.

_____

Chemical Reactions

1. For each example of an equation representing a chemical reaction, indicate whether it is synthesis, decomposition, single replacement, or double replacement, and write the formulas for the reactants and products.

Equation: $H_2CO_3 \rightarrow H_2O + CO_2$
              carbonic acid

Type of reaction:

Reactants:

Products:

Equation: $N_2 + 3H_2 \rightarrow 2NH_3$

Type of reaction:

Reactants:

Products:

Equation: $MgCl_2 + 2NaOH \rightarrow Mg(OH)_2 + 2NaCl$
                                        milk of magnesia

Type of reaction:

Reactants:

Products:

Equation: $C_7H_6O_3 + C_2H_4O_2 \rightarrow C_9H_8O_4 + H_2O$
               salicylic   acetic   aspirin
                 acid   acid

Type of reaction:

Reactants:

Products:

2. In _____ reactions, there is more energy stored in the reactants than in the products. Energy is released in these reactions. Reactions that need an input of energy are called _____ reactions.

3. For each of the following changes, indicate whether the reaction rate will increase (I) or decrease (D).

   A. _____ Grind up the reactants   D. _____ Dilute one reactant

   B. _____ Add a catalyst   E. _____ Cool the reaction mixture

   C. _____ Use more concentrated solutions F. _____ Increase the temperature

4. What is the meaning of the double arrow in the following equation?

   $CO_2 + H_2O \rightleftharpoons H^+ + HCO_3^-$

Mixtures, Solutions, and Suspensions

1. When salt is dissolved in water, the water is called the (a) solution, (b) solute, (c) solvent, (d) liquid, (e) dialysate.

2. Solutions (a) are clear, (b) have a fixed composition, (c) settle when left standing, (d) must be separated by chemical means.

3. Indicate whether each of the following combinations is most accurately described as a mixture, solution, or suspension.

    A. _____ Sugar and salt

    B. _____ Blood cells and plasma

    C. _____ Sugar and water

    D. _____ Cytoplasm of the cell

    E. _____ Sand and water

Acids, Bases, and Buffers

1. Substances that form ions in solution are called _____.

2. Indicate whether each of the following phrases refers to an acid or to a base.

    A. _____ Accepts hydrogen ions

    B. _____ Reacts with a buffer to form a weak acid

    C. _____ Has a sour taste

    D. _____ Reacts with OH⁻ ions to form water

    E. _____ Has a pH of 3.5

    F. _____ Has a slippery, soapy feeling

    G. _____ Donates protons

    H. _____ Has a pH of 8.7

3. Acetic acid ($HC_2H_3O_2$) and sodium acetate ($NaC_2H_3O_2$) are members of a buffer pair. (A) Which member of the buffer pair reacts to neutralize sodium hydroxide (NaOH), and what neutral product is formed? (B) Which member of the buffer pair reacts to neutralize hydrochloric acid (HCl), and what neutral product is formed?

Organic Compounds

1. Carbohydrates contain the elements _____, _____, and _____.

2. Three important hexose monosaccharides are _____, _____, and _____.

3. When two monosaccharides are joined by chemical bonds, the resulting molecule is called a _____.

4. Starch, cellulose, and glycogen are examples of a group of carbohydrates called _____.

16

5. Write the term that is described by each of the following phrases.

A. _____ Element, in addition to C, H, and O, found in all proteins

B. _____ Building blocks of proteins

C. _____ Amino acids that cannot be synthesized in the body

6. Name the following items that pertain to lipids.

A. _____ The building blocks of triglycerides

B. _____ Fatty acids that contain all single covalent bonds

C. _____ Lipids that are an important component of cell membranes

7. Write the term that matches each of the following phrases in the spaces at the left.

A. _____ Forms the genetic material of the cell

B. _____ Single-stranded nucleic acid involved in protein synthesis

C. _____ Building units of nucleic acids

D. _____ Sugar in DNA molecules

E. _____ Double-stranded nucleic acids

F. _____ Five elements in nucleic acids

G. _____ Nucleic acid that contains uracil

H. _____ High-energy compound; contains three phosphate groups

8. Match the following substances with the correct class of organic compounds.

a. carbohydrates   b. lipids   c. proteins   d. nucleic acids

A. _____ Glucose   F. _____ Glycogen

B. _____ Amino acids   G. _____ Hemoglobin

C. _____ Steroids   H. _____ RNA

D. _____ Nucleotides   I. _____ Disaccharides

E. _____ Glycerol   J. _____ Triglycerides

1. On the periodic table in Figure 2-1, use red to color the boxes for the elements that are essential to life.

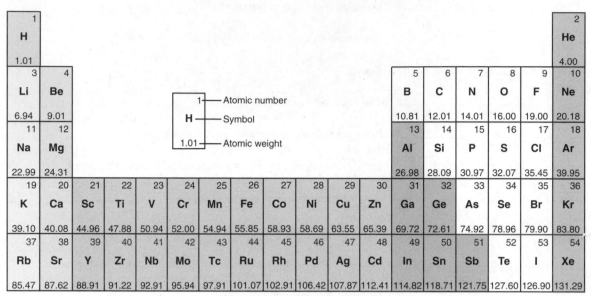

Figure 2-1   Periodic table.

2. Figure 2-2 shows diagrams of six elements in the body. Write the name of the element on the line below the diagram. Use the periodic table in Figure 2-1 to help you identify the elements. Color the nucleus red for hydrogen and oxygen. Color the nucleus blue for carbon and nitrogen. Color the nucleus yellow for sodium and chlorine.

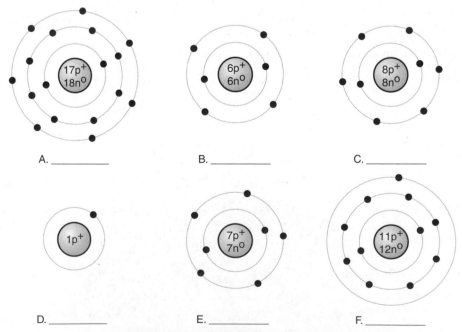

A. _____   B. _____   C. _____

D. _____   E. _____   F. _____

Figure 2-2   Diagrams of elements.

3. Figure 2-3 shows an arrow that represents the pH scale. The line in the center represents a neutral pH. Color the acid portion of the scale red and use blue for the alkaline portion.

4. Which end, A or B, has more hydrogen ions?

5. What is the neutral pH?

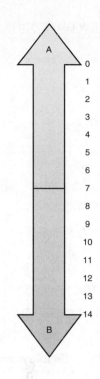

Figure 2-3   pH scale.

6. Figure 2-4 represents the essential amino acid valine. Color the acid group red and the amino group blue. What is the molecular formula for valine?

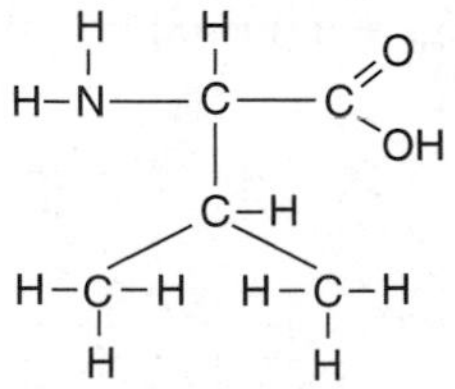

Figure 2-4   Structural formula for valine.

7. Figure 2-5 represents a chain of five nucleotides. Color the phosphates yellow, the nitrogenous bases blue, and the sugars red. Circle each of the five nucleotides.

   A. If this is from DNA, what is the sugar?

   B. What are the four bases in DNA?

   C. What is the sugar in RNA?

   D. What are the four bases in RNA?

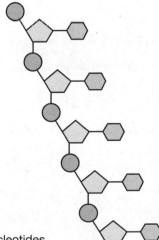

Figure 2-5   Chain of five nucleotides.

REVIEW QUESTIONS

1. What is matter? _____
_____

2. What is the simplest form of matter? _____
_____

3. What is the chemical symbol for (a) oxygen; (b) nitrogen; (c) calcium; (d) potassium; (e) sodium; (f) iron?

    A. Oxygen _____   D. Potassium _____

    B. Nitrogen _____   E. Sodium _____

    C. Calcium _____   F. Iron _____

4. What component of an atom has

    A. a neutral charge?   _____

    B. a negative charge?   _____

    C. negligible mass?   _____

    D. a positive charge?   _____

    E. a mass of one unit?   _____

5. Draw a simplified diagram of a neutral atom that has 11 protons and 12 neutrons.

6. If an atom has 17 protons and 18 neutrons,

    A. What is the mass number?   _____

    B. What is the atomic number?   _____

7. How many electrons are in the highest energy level of the most stable atoms?   _____

8. How does an isotope differ from other atoms of the same element?   _____
_____

9. What is the difference between an ionic bond and a covalent bond?   _____
_____

10. What are *cations* and *anions*?   _____
_____

11. What is a compound, and what is the smallest unit of a compound? _____

_____

_____

12. The molecular formula for sodium bicarbonate is $NaHCO_3$.

    A. What elements are in this compound? _____

    B. How many atoms of each element are present? _____

13. Given the following equation:

$$C_6H_{12}O_6 \;+\; 6O_2 \;\rightarrow\; 6CO_2 \;+\; 6H_2O$$

    A. What are the reactants? _____

    B. What are the products? _____

14. Identify the type of reaction that is represented by each of the following equations:

    A. $S \;+\; O_2 \;\rightarrow\; SO_2$ _____

    B. $Zn \;+\; CuSO_4 \;\rightarrow\; ZnSO_4 \;+\; Cu$ _____

    C. $2NaClO_3 \;\rightarrow\; 2NaCl \;+\; 3O_2$ _____

    D. $HgCl_2 \;+\; H_2S \;\rightarrow\; HgS \;+\; 2HCl$ _____

15. Is the following reaction exergonic or endergonic?

$$ATP \;\rightarrow\; ADP \;+\; P \;+\; energy$$ _____

16. A chemical reaction is proceeding very slowly. Suggest four things you might try to speed up the reaction.

_____

_____

17. The following reaction is reversible:

$$CO_2 \;+\; H_2O \;\rightleftharpoons\; H^+ \;+\; HCO_3^-$$

As you breathe, you exhale CO_2 and remove it from the body. What effect does this have on the above reaction? Does the reaction proceed to the right or to the left as a result of exhaling CO_2?

_____

_____

18. What is the difference between a compound and a mixture?

_____

_____

19. What is the difference between a solution and a suspension?

_____

_____

20. What is an electrolyte? Name two common tests (or graphic tracings) based on electrolyte activity in the body.

_____

_____

21. What is the difference between an acid and a base?

_____

_____

22. What are the reactants and products in a neutralization reaction?

_____

_____

23. What is the pH range of acids? of bases?

_____

_____

24. What are the two components of a buffer solution and what is their purpose?

_____

_____

_____

25. List the five major types of organic compounds that are important in the human body.

_____

_____

26. Give examples and state the importance of three hexose monosaccharides, three disaccharides, and three polysaccharides.

Monosaccharides _____

_____

_____

Disaccharides _____

_____

Polysaccharides _____

_____

27. Describe the structure of proteins.

_____

_____

28. Describe the structure of triglycerides. What is the difference between saturated and unsaturated triglycerides?

_____

_____

_____

29. How do phospholipids and steroids differ from triglycerides?

_____

_____

30. What are three structural differences between the two types of nucleic acids?

_____

_____

_____

VOCABULARY PRACTICE

For each of the following terms, circle the root and write the definition of the root in the space provided.

1. aerobic _____   6. lactose _____

2. hyperbaric _____   7. calorimeter _____

3. endergonic _____   8. alkalosis _____

4. hydrotherapy _____   9. pentolysis _____

5. lipogenesis _____   10. saccharide _____

11. For each of the following terms, circle the prefix and write the definition of the prefix in the space provided.

A. exergonic _____   F. triceps _____

B. diatomic _____   G. mononuclear _____

C. unicellular _____   H. abduct _____

D. tetrachloride _____   I. hexagonal _____

E. polyplegia _____   J. endergonic _____

12. For each of the following terms, circle the suffix and write the definition of the suffix in the space provided.

A. diuresis _____   F. hydrolysis _____

B. glycogenesis _____   G. calorimeter _____

C. nephroptosis _____   H. physiologist _____

D. pentose _____   I. cardiology _____

E. chloride _____   J. pharyngitis _____

13. Match the definitions on the left with the correct clinical term from the column on the right by placing the corresponding letter in the space before the definition.

A. _____ Nonproprietary drug name assigned by the USAN council

B. _____ Presence of a disease in a given population at all times

C. _____ Study of causes of diseases

D. _____ Alpha-methyl-4(2 methylpropyl) benzene

E. _____ An illness that occurs without any known cause

F. _____ Smallest unit is a molecule

G. _____ Drug name that is assigned by the manufacturing company

H. _____ An infection acquired from the place of treatment

I. _____ The water in a normal saline solution

J. _____ A widespread epidemic; occurs over a large geographical area

1. Brand name
2. Chemical name
3. Compound
4. Endemic
5. Etiology
6. Generic name
7. Idiopathic
8. Nosocomial
9. Pandemic
10. Solvent

14. Write the meaning of each of the following clinical abbreviations.

A. CHO _____

B. VS _____

C. ADL _____

D. stat _____

E. Rx _____

F. DNR _____

G. ECF _____

H. ICU _____

I. NA _____

J. ad lib _____

15. Spelling is important in scientific and medical applications because only one or two incorrect letters can change the meaning. Six of the following words from this chapter are misspelled. Place a check mark (✓) in the space if it is spelled correctly. Write the correct spelling in the space if it is spelled incorrectly.

A. proteen _____

B. asid _____

C. covalent _____

D. element _____

E. iatrogenic _____

F. akalosis _____

G. colliodal _____

H. deoxyribose _____

I. hydrogenated _____

J. disackharide _____

16. Using word parts from this chapter, write words that have the following meanings.

A. Requires air or oxygen _____

B. Characterized by greater than normal pressure _____

24

Chapter **2** **Chemistry, Matter, and Life**

C. Production of fat _____

D. Oxygen combined with hemoglobin _____

E. Capable of taking apart sugar _____

TESTING COMPREHENSION

1. The chemical symbol for the element carbon is (a) Cu, (b) C, (c) Ca, (d) Co.

2. The chemical symbol for the element iron is (a) Fe, (b) I, (c) P, (d) Cu.

3. If a neutral atom has a mass number of 35 and has 17 electrons, what is the atomic number of this atom? (a) 35, (b) 18, (c) 52, (d) 17.

4. The mass number of a atom equals the (a) number of protons in the nucleus, (b) number of electrons in the energy shells, (c) number of protons plus the number of neutrons, (d) number of neutrons plus electrons.

5. A radioactive isotope of iodine has (a) more electrons than normal iodine, (b) more protons than normal iodine, (c) more neutrons than normal iodine, (d) more energy shells than normal iodine.

6. Two atoms of hydrogen share their electrons to form a molecule of hydrogen gas. This is an example of a (a) hydrogen bond, (b) covalent bond, (c) ionic bond, (d) intermolecular bond.

7. The molecular formula for sodium bicarbonate is $NaHCO_3$. How many atoms are in a molecule of sodium bicarbonate? (a) 6; (b) 4; (c) 3; (d) 2.

8. What type of chemical reaction is represented by the following equation:

   $$Zn + CuSO_4 \rightarrow ZnSO_4 + Cu$$

   (a) synthesis, (b) decomposition, (c) single replacement, (d) double replacement.

9. Human blood has a normal pH = 7.4. This means that it is (a) slightly acidic, (b) slightly alkaline, (c) strongly acidic, (d) strongly alkaline.

10. Given the neutralization reaction $NaOH + HCl \rightarrow NaCl + H_2O$, what is the acid? (a) NaOH, (b) HCl, (c) NaCl, (d) H_2O.

11. Assume that a reaction is proceeding at a given rate. Which of the following will decrease the reaction rate? (a) add a catalyst, (b) crush the reactants into smaller particles, (c) increase the concentration of the reactants, (d) decrease the temperature.

12. Which of the following pairs of compounds are both monosaccharides? (a) galactose and lactose, (b) cellulose and glycogen, (c) glucose and maltose, (d) glucose and fructose.

13. Common table sugar is sucrose. Sucrose has (a) more carbon atoms than fructose, (b) more carbon atoms than glycogen, (c) more carbon atoms than cellulose, (d) more carbon atoms than maltose.

14. The storage form of carbohydrates in the body is (a) cellulose, (b) glycogen, (c) starch, (d) glucose.

15. The element that is present in proteins but is not present in carbohydrates is (a) carbon, (b) hydrogen, (c) nitrogen, (d) oxygen.

16. Which of the following pertain to lipids? (a) triglycerides and fatty acids, (b) peptide bonds and amino acids, (c) adenine and cytosine, (d) amino acids and fatty acids.

17. A nucleotide molecule consists of (a) adenine and guanine; (b) a sugar, nitrogenous base, and a phosphate; (c) glucose, adenine, and a nitrogenous base; (d) a phosphate, deoxyribose, and glucose.

18. Ribose and deoxyribose are (a) pentose sugars, (b) nitrogenous bases, (c) hexose sugars, (d) polysaccharides.

19. What nitrogenous base is present in RNA, but is not in DNA? (a) adenine, (b) guanine, (c) uracil, (d) thymine.

20. Which of the following is **not** true about nucleic acids? (a) DNA consists of two strands; (b) both DNA and RNA contain nucleotides; (c) RNA functions in protein synthesis; (d) both DNA and RNA contain thymine.

21. Which of the following best describes ATP? (a) it is part of a buffer system to neutralize acids, (b) it is a compound that has high energy bonds between phosphate atoms, (c) it is a radioactive isotope of phosphate, (d) it is an intermediate molecule in the conversion of DNA to RNA.

22. Sara acquired a nosocomial infection. This type of illness (a) is present within a given population at all times, (b) has no known cause, (c) is acquired from the place of treatment, (d) has no detectable physical changes to explain the symptoms.

23. Lori decided she wanted to be an etiologist. To do this, she would spend many years (a) studying the causes of disease, (b) studying illnesses that occur without any known cause, (c) studying endemic diseases, (d) studying idiopathic disorders.

24. Jon was studying endergonic reactions in chemistry class. His teacher explained that (a) there is more energy stored in the product than in the reactants in these reactions, (b) there is more energy on the left side of the equation than on the right in these reactions, (c) the conversion of ATP to ADP is this type of reaction, (d) these reactions require high pressures of oxygen.

25. Jacob performed experiments using a calorimeter. He was studying (a) changes in oxygen pressure, (b) changes in heat energy, (c) changes in muscle tension, (d) changes in voltage during heart contractions.

A STEP BEYOND

Go a step beyond the ordinary and learn more about a topic that is related to this chapter but not discussed in detail in the textbook. Select one of the following topics, or one suggested by your instructor, and write a brief paper (250 words minimum), create a poster, or develop a short presentation (approximately 4 to 5 minutes) that focuses on your selection. Suggested topics for this chapter include the following:

1. *Radioactive isotopes*. Learn about the use of radioactive isotopes in medicine. You may choose either diagnostic use or therapeutic use. Also, you may focus on one isotope with more depth or do a summary of several isotopes.

2. *Types of radiation*. Learn the differences between alpha, beta, and gamma radiation. Include the nature of each type and the effects they have on the body.

3. *Lead poisoning*. A lot of attention is given to lead poisoning. What is it? What are some common sources? How does it affect the body? Why does it act as poison?

Word Scramble

Determine the word that fits each definition; then write the word in the spaces below the definition, one letter per space. The letters in the boxes form a scrambled word. Unscramble the letters to create a word that matches the final definition in each section.

1. Smallest unit of a compound

2. Positively charged subatomic particle

3. Building block of a protein

4. Accepts protons

5. Product in a neutralization reaction

6. Speeds up a chemical reaction

7. One of the elements in water

8. A complex carbohydrate

Letters to use for final words: _____

Final definition: High-energy compound

_____

9. An element in water

10. Sugar in RNA

11. Element always present in proteins

12. Group of compounds that includes fats

13. A hexose monosaccharide

14. Positively charged ion

15. Negatively charged subatomic particle

16. Resists change in pH

17. Fat with three fatty acids

Letters to use for final words: _____

Final definition: Genetic material of the cell

_____

3 Cell Structure and Function

Structure of the Generalized Cell

1. List five functions of the various proteins that are found in the cell membrane.

   A. _____

   B. _____

   C. _____

   D. _____

   E. _____

2. The following phrases refer to the cell membrane. Write the term that applies to each descriptive phrase.

   A. _____   Two main structural components of the membrane

   _____

   B. _____   Center of the membrane

   C. _____   Outside and inside layers of the membrane

   D. _____   Reaction of lipid to water

   E. _____   Reaction of phosphate to water

3. The following phrases refer to the inside of the cell, the region inside the membrane. Write the term that applies to each descriptive phase.

   A. _____   Gel-like fluid inside the cell

   B. _____   Structures that have specific roles in metabolism inside the cell

   C. _____   Water component of cytoplasm

   D. _____   Bodies that are temporarily inside the cell

   E. _____   Control center for metabolic activities inside the cell

4. Name the cellular component described by each of the following phrases.

A. _____ Contains enzymes for production of adenosine triphosphate (ATP)

B. _____ Contains digestive enzymes

C. _____ Prepares products for exocytosis

D. _____ Granules of RNA in the cytoplasm

E. _____ Located in the centrosome

F. _____ Propels substances across the surface of the cell

G. _____ Membranous transport system within the cell

H. _____ Long strands of DNA within the nucleus

I. _____ Functions to move the cell

J. _____ Dark structure that contains RNA in the nucleus

K. _____ Semiliquid around the organelles

L. _____ Controls flow of materials into and out of the cell

M. _____ Organelle that controls cell functions

N. _____ Forms the cytoskeleton (two answers)

_____

Cell Functions

1. Indicate whether each of the following refers to simple diffusion, facilitated diffusion, osmosis, or filtration.

A. _____ Movement of water through a selectively permeable membrane

B. _____ Movement of gases into the lungs

C. _____ Requires a carrier molecule

2. Identify each of the following transport mechanisms as active transport, passive transport, endocytosis, or exocytosis.

A. _____ Utilizes ATP and a carrier molecule

B. _____ Phagocytosis

C. _____ Osmosis

D. _____ Releases secretory products through the cell membrane

E. _____ Transports ions from low to high concentrations

F. _____ Facilitated diffusion

G. _____ Incorporates fluid droplets into the cytoplasm

3. The accompanying diagram represents two solutions separated by a selectively permeable membrane. Answer the following questions about these solutions.

Solution A 5%	Solution B 1%

_____ Which solution is hypertonic?

_____ Which solution will increase in volume because of osmosis?

4. Each of the following phrases refers to an event during the cell cycle. Write the state of event that is described by each phrase.

A. _____ Period between active cell divisions

B. _____ Chromosomes align along center of cell

C. _____ Cytokinesis occurs

D. _____ DNA and centrioles replicate

E. _____ Spindle fibers form

F. _____ Nuclear membrane reforms

G. _____ Chromatin shortens and thickens

H. _____ Chromosomes move toward centrioles

5. Compare *mitosis* and *meiosis* by answering the questions in the following table.

	Mitosis	Meiosis
In what type of cell does each occur?		
How many new cells are produced in each completed division?		
If the original cell has 46 chromosomes (23 pairs), how many are in each new cell?		

6. A neoplasm develops when _____ is uncontrolled.

7. The following is a sequence of bases in a portion of the gene that codes for the human hormone oxytocin.

   A = adenine   C = cytosine   G = guanine   T = thymine   U = uracil

   T A C A C A A T G T A A G T T T T G

   A. Write out the sequence of bases on the corresponding mRNA molecule and mark off the codons on the molecule.

   _____

   B. Write out the sequence of bases on the six anticodons on the tRNA molecules.

   _____

LABELING AND COLORING EXERCISES

1. Identify the parts of the generalized cell in the Figure 3-1 by placing the correct letter in the space provided by the listed labels. Then select different colors for each structure and use them to color the coding circles and the corresponding structures in the illustration.

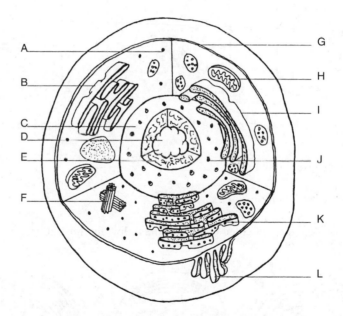

Figure 3-1   Diagram of a generalized cell.

_____ Cell membrane ○	_____ Golgi apparatus ○	_____ Nucleus ○
_____ Centriole ○	_____ Mitochondria ○	_____ Ribosome ○
_____ Chromatin ○	_____ Nuclear pore ○	_____ RER ○
_____ Cilia ○	_____ Nucleolus ○	_____ SER ○

Chapter **3 Cell Structure and Function**

2. Figure 3-2 shows a section of the cell membrane. Color the phosphate blue, proteins yellow, and the lipid portion pink. Identify the hydrophilic area and the hydrophobic area.

INTRACELLULAR AREA

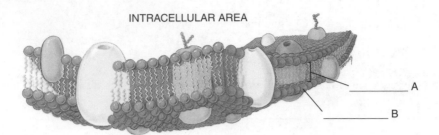

_____ A

_____ B

Figure 3-2   Structure of the cell membrane.

3. Figure 3-3 shows a red blood cell in three different solutions. Color the hypertonic solution yellow and the hypotonic solution pink. Leave the isotonic solution uncolored.

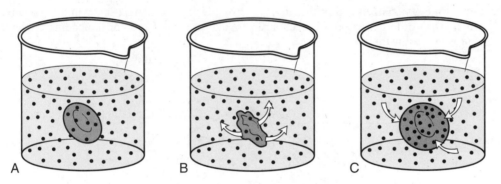

A   B   C

Figure 3-3   Effects of three different solutions on red blood cells.

Which solution, A, B, or C, causes crenation? _____

Which solution, A, B, or C, causes hemolysis? _____

4. Identify the phase of mitosis that is represented by each of the following illustrations.

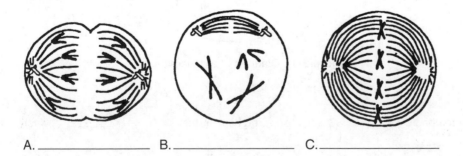

A. _____   B. _____   C. _____

REVIEW QUESTIONS

1. What is a generalized or composite cell?

   _____

   _____

2. What are the two major types of molecules in the cell membrane? How are they arranged?

   _____

   _____

3. What are the functions of the proteins in the cell membrane?

   _____

   _____

   _____

4. What is the gel-like fluid inside the cell?

   _____

5. Describe chromatin and the nucleolus. Tell where they are located, the major components, and functions of each.

   _____

   _____

   _____

6. What is the structure and function of each of the following cytoplasmic organelles? (a) mitochondria, (b) ribosomes, (c) rough endoplasmic reticulum, (d) smooth endoplasmic reticulum, (e) Golgi apparatus, (f) lysosomes

   _____

   _____

   _____

7. What two types of protein structures form the cytoskeleton?

   _____

8. Where are the centrioles located and what is their function?

   _____

   _____

9. What are three differences between cilia and flagella?

   _____

   _____

10. List the parts of a cell.

A. _____

B. _____

C. _____

D. _____

E. _____

F. _____

G. _____

H. _____

I. _____

J. _____

K. _____

L. _____

11. What role does the cell membrane have in determining the composition of the cytoplasm?

_____

_____

12. Illustrate the process of diffusion by describing a physiologic example.

_____

_____

13. How is facilitated diffusion different from simple diffusion? In what ways are the two processes alike?

_____

_____

14. Describe the conditions under which osmosis occurs.

_____

_____

15. Describe what will happen to a red blood cell when it is placed in (a) an isotonic solution, (b) a hypertonic solution, (c) a hypotonic solution.

_____

_____

_____

16. Describe the conditions under which filtration occurs.

_____

_____

17. State two ways in which active transport is different from facilitated diffusion. State two ways in which they are similar.

_____

_____

18. What is the difference between endocytosis and exocytosis? What is the difference between phagocytosis and pinocytosis?

_____

_____

19. Describe each of the following:

A. interphase _____

_____

_____

B. prophase _____

_____

_____

C. metaphase _____

_____

_____

D. anaphase _____

_____

_____

E. telophase _____

_____

_____

20. If you start with one cell that has 46 chromosomes,

A. How many cells will you have after one complete mitotic division? _____

B. How many chromosomes will be in each cell after mitosis? _____

C. How many cells will you have after one complete division by meiosis? _____

D. How many chromosomes will be in each cell after meiosis? _____

21. How do neoplasms develop?

_____

22. What are genes and where are they located?

_____

_____

23. What are the complementary base pairs in DNA? What is their role in DNA replication?

_____

_____

24. What is the difference between mRNA and tRNA? What role does each one have in protein synthesis?

_____

_____

_____

25. Transcription and translation both occur in protein synthesis. Describe each of these processes.

_____

_____

_____

VOCABULARY PRACTICE

Match the definitions on the left with the correct clinical term from the column on the right by placing the corresponding number in the space before the definition.

1. _____ Loss of differentiation of cells; characteristic of cancer

2. _____ The route used when administering medications by intravenous, intramuscular, or intradermal injections

3. _____ Red blood cells shrink when placed in a hypertonic solution; an example of this transport process

4. _____ Enlargement of an organ due to increase in size of constituent cells

5. _____ Process by which a cell may engulf bacteria

6. _____ Death of a group of cells

7. _____ Any new or abnormal growth; tumor

8. _____ It takes cellular energy to move sodium from low to high concentration in the kidney; an example of this transport process

9. _____ Not malignant; not recurring

10. _____ Type of cell division that produces sperm

A. Active transport
B. Anaplasia
C. Benign
D. Hyperplasia
E. Hypertrophy
F. Meiosis
G. Mitosis
H. Necrosis
I. Neoplasm
J. Osmosis
K. Parenteral
L. Percutaneous
M. Phagocytosis
N. Pinocytosis

11. Write the meaning of each of the following clinical abbreviations.

A. DNA _____

B. MRI _____

C. LBW _____

D. NB _____

E. NPO _____

12. Spelling is important in scientific and medical applications because only one or two incorrect letters can change the meaning. Three of the following words from this chapter are misspelled. Place a check mark (✓) in the space before the word if it is spelled correctly. Write the correct spelling in the space if it is spelled incorrectly.

A. benine _____

B. anomoly _____

C. meiosis _____

D. cytokinesis _____

E. displasis _____

13. Some of the following words may have more than one root. In all cases, give the meaning of the *first* root that appears in the word.

A. cytoplasm _____   F. etiology _____

B. phagocytosis _____   G. hiatus _____

C. hypertonic _____   H. dysphagia _____

D. somatic _____   I. pinocytosis _____

E. reticulum _____   J. quadriceps _____

14. Underline the suffix in each of the following words and write the meaning of the suffix on the line following the word.

A. hydrophilic _____   F. colostomy _____

B. organelle _____   G. venule _____

C. scoliosis _____   H. pericardium _____

D. cellulitis _____   I. anatomist _____

E. pericardial _____   J. colonoscopy _____

15. Write words that fit the following definitions

   A. Wasting away; a decrease in size _____

   B. An agent that causes cancer _____

   C. Study of cells _____

   D. Transformation of one cell type into another _____

   E. Spread of a tumor to a secondary site _____

   F. Death of cells _____

   G. New or abnormal growth _____

   H. Outside the cell _____

   I. Difficulty in eating or swallowing _____

   J. Pertaining to the body _____

TESTING COMPREHENSION

1. The cell (plasma) membrane is composed primarily of (a) phospholipid and proteins, (b) proteins and carbohydrates, (c) lipid and carbohydrate, (d) phosphate and carbohydrate.

2. The portion of the cell membrane that is hydrophobic is (a) phosphate, (b) protein, (c) lipid, (d) carbohydrate.

3. Mitochondria in a cell function (a) to package secretory products, (b) in energy production, (c) to produce spindle fibers, (d) in the transport of substances within the cell.

4. Ribosomes (a) are attached to the cristae of mitochondria, (b) function is protein synthesis, (c) function to transfer genetic information from the nucleus to the cytoplasm, (d) are found in the nucleus of the cell.

5. A selectively permeable membrane permits (a) diffusion but not osmosis; (b) filtration but not diffusion or osmosis; (c) unrestricted movement of water and solutes; (d) certain, but not all, substances to enter and leave the cell.

6. Which of the following is **incorrect** about cellular organelles? (a) most ATP is produced in the mitochondria; (b) lysosomes contain digestive enzymes; (c) Golgi apparatus produces DNA; (d) ribosomes function in protein synthesis.

7. During which stage of mitosis do chromosomes move away from the center of the cell? (a) prophase, (b) telophase, (c) metaphase, (d) anaphase.

8. During which stage of mitosis does the DNA replicate? (a) prophase, (b) interphase, (c) telophase, (d) metaphase.

9. Short hairlike structures on the surface of some cells are (a) flagella, (b) protein channels, (c) cilia, (d) secretory vacuoles.

10. Two solutions of equal volume are separated by a selectively permeable membrane that is permeable to the solvent but not permeable to the solute. Solution A is a 0.9% glucose and solution B is a 5% glucose. When equilibrium is established after osmosis, (a) solution A will have decreased volume and increased concentration; (b) solution A will have decreased volume and decreased concentration; (c) solution A will have increased volume and increased concentration; (d) solution A will have increased volume and decreased concentration.

11. Which one of the following does **not** move solutes from a region of higher concentration to a region of lower concentration? (a) simple diffusion, (b) facilitated diffusion, (c) osmosis, (d) positive transport.

12. Which one of the following uses cellular energy? (a) simple diffusion, (b) active transport, (c) facilitated diffusion, (d) osmosis.

13. When a red blood cell is placed in a hypotonic solution, the cell will (a) shrink, (b) swell, (c) crenate, (d) dissolve.

14. If a cell has 46 chromosomes, (a) there will be four cells, each with 23 chromosomes after mitosis; (b) there will be four cells, each with 46 chromosomes after mitosis; (c) there will be two cells, each with 23 chromosomes after mitosis; (d) there will be two cells, each with 46 chromosomes after mitosis.

15. In DNA replication, (a) adenine always pairs with thymine; (b) adenine always pairs with cytosine; (c) adenine always pairs with guanine; (d) cytosine always pairs with thymine.

16. During transcription, (a) DNA is replicated; (b) tRNA transfers an amino acid to a ribosome; (c) a codon on mRNA pairs with an anticodon on tRNA; (d) genetic information is transferred from DNA to mRNA.

17. A sequence of three bases on mRNA is called (a) an anticodon, (b) gene, (c) an amino acid, (d) a codon.

18. Jason has a congenital disorder. This indicates that (a) it was present at birth; (b) it was caused by a defective gene; (c) it was due to anaplasia; (d) it was malignant.

19. An increase in the number of cells due to an increase in the frequency of cell division is called (a) hypertrophy, (b) metaplasia, (c) atrophy, (d) hyperplasia.

20. The death of a group of cells is called (a) atrophy, (b) necrosis, (c) neoplasm, (d) dysplasia.

21. Let A = adenine, C = cytosine, G = guanine, T = thymine, and U = uracil. If a sequence on DNA is TAG, the complementary sequence on MRNA after transcription is (a) ATC, (b) TAG, (c) AUC, (d) UAG.

22. Which one of the following nitrogenous bases is **not** found in DNA? (a) adenine, (b) uracil, (c) guanine, (d) thymine.

23. Anatomy and anaphase have the same root. This root means (a) structure, (b) apart, (c) cell division, (d) pertaining to.

24. Cytokinesis means (a) division of the cytoplasm, (b) division of the cell membrane, (c) division of the chromosomes, (d) division of the nucleus.

25. Which one of the following is **not** made of microtubules? (a) cilia, (b) flagella, (c) centrioles, (d) microvilli.

A STEP BEYOND

Go a step beyond the ordinary and learn more about a topic that is related to this chapter but not discussed in detail in the textbook. Select one of the following topics, or one suggested by your instructor, and write a brief paper (250 words minimum), create a poster, or develop a short presentation (approximately 4 to 5 minutes) that focuses on your selection. Suggested topics for this chapter include the following:

1. *Prokaryotic and eukaryotic cells.* Investigate the differences between these two cell types. Which type of cells do you have? Where is the genetic material in each type?

2. *History of cell biology.* Investigate the early history of cell biology. Learn about the contributions of Antonie van Leeuwenhoek, Robert Hooke, Theodor Schwann and Matthias Jakob Schleiden, Louis Pasteur, and Rudolph Virchow.

3. *Neoplasms*. What are neoplasms? How do they develop? What is the difference between benign and malignant neoplasms? How are neoplasms named?

4. *HeLa cells*. What are HeLa cells? What is their importance? How are they used?

FUN & GAMES

Word Scramble

Determine the word that fits each definition, and then write the word in the spaces below the definition, one letter per space. The letters in the boxes form a scrambled word. Unscramble the letters to create a word that matches the final definition in each section.

1. Wasting away

2. Not malignant

3. Study of cells

4. Diffusion of water through a selectively permeable membrane

5. An agent that causes cancer

Letters to use for final word: _____

Final definition: Cell eating

_____

6. Alteration in size, shape, and organization of cells.

7. Movement from high to low concentration

8. Somatic cell division

9. Division of cytoplasm

Letters to use for final word: _____

Final definition: Cell drinking

_____

4 Tissues and Membranes

LEARNING EXERCISES

Body Tissues

1. Write a sentence that defines the term *tissue*.

   _____

   _____

2. The study of tissues is called _____.

3. List the four types of tissues found in the body.

   _____

   _____

   _____

   _____

4. Complete the description of epithelial tissue by writing the correct words in the blanks.

   Epithelial tissues consist of _____ cells with _____ intercellular matrix. They

   have _____ surface, have no _____ supply, and _____

   quickly. These tissues _____ the body, _____ body cavities, and

   _____ the organs within the body cavities. The cells may be _____,

   _____, or _____ in shape.

5. Match the types of epithelial tissue with their descriptions or locations below. The types of tissue may be used more than once.

   A. _____ Can be stretched in response to tension

   B. _____ Some cells are short and some are tall

   C. _____ Single layer of thin, flat cells

   D. _____ Lining kidney tubules

   E. _____ Many layers

   F. _____ Lining the urinary bladder

   G. _____ Capillary walls

   H. _____ Outer layer of skin

   1. Simple squamous
   2. Stratified squamous
   3. Simple cuboidal
   4. Simple columnar
   5. Pseudostratified columnar
   6. Transitional

I. _____ Found in many glands

J. _____ Height greater than width and depth

K. _____ Often has cilia and goblet cells

L. _____ Alveoli (air sacs) of the lungs

M. _____ May have goblet cells and microvilli

N. _____ Lines the stomach and intestines

O. _____ Lines portions of the respiratory tract

P. _____ Width, depth, and height are equal

6. Write "endocrine" before each phrase that refers to an endocrine gland and write "exocrine" before each phrase that refers to an exocrine gland.

A. _____ Ductless gland

B. _____ Goblet cells

C. _____ Secrete product onto a surface

D. _____ Have ducts

E. _____ Secrete product into blood

7. Match each of the following phrases about glands with the term it best describes. There is one answer for each phrase.

A. _____ Ducts do not have branches

B. _____ Glandular portion is round

C. _____ Entire cell is discharged with secretion

D. _____ No cytoplasm is lost with secretion

E. _____ Portion of cell is lost with secretion

1. compound

2. simple

3. tubular

4. acinar

5. merocrine

6. apocrine

7. holocrine

8. Write the terms that match the following phrases about connective tissue.

A. _____ Fibers that are strong and flexible

B. _____ Connective tissue cells that are phagocytic

C. _____ Type that anchors skin to underlying tissues

D. _____ Type that contains fat

E. _____ Type that is found in tendons and ligaments

F. _____ Covering around cartilage

G. _____ Type of cartilage in intervertebral discs

H. _____ Most rigid connective tissue

I. _____ Structural unit of bone

J. _____ Bone cells

K. _____ Connective tissue with liquid matrix

L. _____ Another name for red blood cells

9. Write the terms that match the following phrases about muscle tissue.

A. _____ Two types of contractile protein fibers in muscle tissue

_____

B. _____ Another name for striated voluntary muscle

C. _____ Muscle in the wall of the stomach

D. _____ Muscle cells are spindle-shaped and tapered

E. _____ Muscle tissue in the heart

F. _____ Muscle tissue in the deltoid muscle of the shoulder

G. _____ Another name for striated involuntary muscle

H. _____ Muscle with branching fibers

I. _____ Has intercalated disks

10. Write the terms that match the following phrases about nervous tissue.

A. _____ Cells that transmit impulses

B. _____ Take impulses to cell body

C. _____ Take impulses away for cell body

D. _____ Supporting cells of nerve tissue

Inflammation and Tissue Repair

1. Which characteristic of inflammation results from

A. blood vessel dilation _____

B. increased vascular permeability _____

Indicate whether each of the following phrases pertains to regeneration (R) or fibrosis (F).

2. _____ Scar tissue

3. _____ Surface abrasions

43

4. _____ Cells identical to original cells

5. _____ Granulation tissue

6. _____ Occurs only in tissues capable of mitosis

7. _____ Occurs in skeletal muscle

8. _____ Proliferation of collagen fibers

Body Membranes

1. Write the terms that match the following phrases about body membranes.

A. _____ Membranes composed only of connective tissue

B. _____ Line cavities that open to the outside

C. _____ Type of membrane lining the digestive tract

D. _____ Membranes with two layers

E. _____ Layer that lines a cavity wall

F. _____ Layer that covers organs within a cavity

G. _____ Serous membrane associated with the lungs

H. _____ Serous membrane associated with the heart

I. _____ Serous membrane of abdominopelvic cavity

J. _____ Connective tissue membrane of movable joints

K. _____ Connective tissue membranes around the brain

L. _____ Tough outermost layer of meninges

M. _____ Middle layer of the meninges

N. _____ Innermost layer of the meninges

LABELING AND COLORING EXERCISES

1. Match the following illustrations of epithelial tissues with the correct tissue type and location. Select your answers from the list provided for you.

Type of Epithelium
Simple squamous
Simple cuboidal
Simple columnar with cilia
Pseudostratified ciliated columnar
Stratified squamous
Transitional

Locations
Digestive tract
Respiratory passages
Urinary bladder
Skin
Alveoli of lungs
Kidneys

A. Type _____

    Location _____

B. Type _____

    Location _____

C. Type _____

    Location _____

2. Answer the following questions about the accompanying diagram.

    A. What type of connective tissue is illustrated in this diagram?

    _____

    B. What type of fiber is represented by letter A?

    _____

    C. What type of fiber is represented by letter B?

    _____

3. Answer the following questions about the accompanying diagram.

    A. What type of connective tissue is illustrated in this diagram?

    _____

    B. What type of protein is found in the intercellular matrix A?

    _____

    C. What is the name of the cell represented by letter B?

    _____

D. What is the space represented by letter C?

_____

4. Answer the following questions about the accompanying diagram.

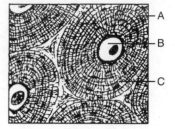

A. What type of connective tissue is illustrated in this diagram?

_____

B. What term is used for the concentric rings of matrix represented by letter A?

_____

C. What is the central structure represented by letter B?

_____

D. What term is used for the tiny hairlike structures represented by letter C?

_____

5. Answer the following questions about the accompanying diagram.

A. What type of muscle tissue is illustrated in this diagram?

_____

B. What term is used for the cell membrane represented by letter A?

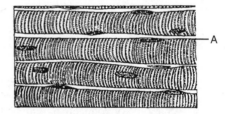

_____

C. What two types of contractile proteins are found in this tissue?

_____

6. Answer the following questions about the accompanying diagram.

A. What type of muscle tissue is illustrated in this diagram?

_____

B. Give two locations for this type of muscle tissue.

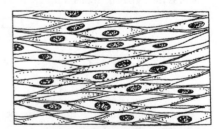

_____

7. Answer the following questions about the accompanying diagram.

A. What type of muscle tissue is illustrated in this diagram?

_____

B. What is the term for the dark band represented by letter B?

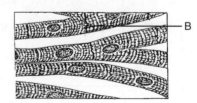

_____

C. Where is this type of muscle located?

_____

1. What constitutes a tissue?

   _____

   _____

2. What is the term given to the microscopic study of tissues?

   _____

3. Name the four main types of tissues found in the body.

   _____   _____

   _____   _____

4. List five functions of epithelial tissues and tell where these tissues are located.

   _____

   _____

   _____

   _____

5. Which item in each of the following pairs of items refers to epithelial tissue?

   A. relatively large amount of matrix; relatively small amount of matrix

   B. poor mitotic capabilities; readily mitotic

   C. abundant blood supply; has no blood vessels

   D. closely packed cells; scattered cells

   E. always surrounded by other tissues; always has a free surface

6. What is the difference between simple epithelium and stratified epithelium?

   _____

   _____

   _____

7. Describe the appearance of each of the following:

   A. simple squamous epithelium   _____

   B. simple columnar epithelium   _____

   C. pseudostratified columnar epithelium   _____

   D. stratified squamous epithelium   _____

47

8. Indicate where each of the following is found:

   A. simple cuboidal epithelium   _____

   B. simple columnar epithelium   _____

   C. transitional epithelium   _____

   D. stratified squamous epithelium   _____

9. What is the difference between exocrine and endocrine glands?

_____

_____

_____

10. What type of gland are goblet cells?

_____

11. What is the difference in shape between tubular glands and alveolar glands?

_____

_____

12. What is the difference among merocrine, apocrine, and holocrine glands?

_____

_____

_____

13. Compare the structural features of connective tissue with the structural features of epithelial tissue.

_____

_____

_____

14. Describe the characteristics of collagenous fibers and elastic fibers.

_____

_____

15. What is the function of each of the following cells: fibroblast, macrophage, mast cell?

_____

_____

_____

16. What is another name for loose connective tissue? Where is it found?

_____

17. How does dense fibrous connective tissue differ from loose connective tissue? Where is dense fibrous connective tissue located?

_____

_____

18. Use the following terms in a description of cartilage: chondrin, chondrocytes, lacunae, perichondrium.

_____

_____

_____

19. What is the difference in structure between hyaline cartilage, fibrocartilage, and elastic cartilage? Where is each type located?

_____

_____

_____

20. Use the following terms in a description of the structure of osseous tissue: osteon, haversian canal, lamellae, osteocytes, lacunae, canaliculi.

_____

_____

_____

_____

21. What is the term for each of the following?

A. red blood cells _____

B. white blood cells _____

C. platelets _____

D. intercellular matrix _____

22. What are actin and myosin?

_____

23. Indicate whether each of the following pertains to skeletal muscle, smooth muscle, or cardiac muscle.

A. multinucleated _____

B. intercalated disks _____

C. spindle-shaped cells _____

D. cross-striations

_____

E. located in the wall of internal organs

_____

F. under voluntary control

_____

24. What is the difference between neurons and neuroglia?

_____

_____

25. Use the terms *axon, dendrite,* and *cell body* in a description of the neuron.

_____

_____

_____

26. What are the characteristics and benefits of inflammation?

_____

_____

27. What are the two types of tissue repair and which one produces scar tissue?

_____

_____

28. What is the difference in structure between epithelial membranes and connective tissue membranes?

_____

_____

29. Where are mucous membranes located?

_____

_____

_____

30. Where are serous membranes located?

_____

_____

31. Describe the specific location for each of the following:

A. parietal pleura

_____

B. visceral pericardium

_____

C. parietal peritoneum

_____

32. What type of membrane is described by each of the following?

   A. lines joint cavities _____

   B. surrounds the brain and spinal cord _____

   C. one layer is the dura mater _____

VOCABULARY PRACTICE

Match the definitions on the left with the correct term from the column on the right by placing the corresponding number in the space before the definition. Not all terms will be used.

1. _____ Study that involves the absorption and distribution of a drug

2. _____ Tumor derived from fat cells

3. _____ Abnormal joining of tissues by scar tissue

4. _____ Cells that release histamine in allergic reactions

5. _____ Removal and microscopic examination of tissues

6. _____ Study of the structural and functional changes in tissues caused by disease

7. _____ Malignant growth derived from connective tissue cells

8. _____ Malignant growth derived from epithelial cells

A. Adhesion
B. Biopsy
C. Carcinoma
D. Lipoma
E. Macrophage
F. Mast cell
G. Pathology
H. Pharmacodynamics
I. Pharmacokinetics
J. Sarcoma

9. Write the meaning of the following abbreviations.

   A. PMH _____   F. cath _____

   B. NS _____   G. ac _____

   C. IM _____   H. OD _____

   D. LPN _____   I. PO _____

   E. ASA _____   J. pc _____

10. Spelling is important in scientific and medical applications because only one or two incorrect letters can change the meaning. Four of the following words from this chapter are misspelled. Place a check mark (✓) in the space before the word if it is spelled correctly. Write the correct spelling in the space if it is spelled incorrectly.

   A. skurvy _____   F. rithrosite _____

   B. macrophage _____   G. skwaymus _____

   C. condrocte _____   H. myoma _____

   D. neuroglia _____   I. myosin _____

   E. papilloma _____   J. epithelium _____

11. For each of the following words, underline the root and write the meaning of the root on the line following the word.

A. vacuous _____   E. adipose _____

B. auscultation _____   F. stratified _____

C. cohesive _____   G. inoculation _____

D. stricture _____

12. Write the meaning of the underlined portion of the following words of the line following each word.

A. macrophage _____   F. adenoma _____

B. pseudostratified _____   G. neuroglia _____

C. multinuclear _____   H. neuroglia _____

D. osteoblast _____   I. erythrocyte _____

E. carcinoma _____   J. squamous _____

13. From your knowledge of word parts, write words that have the following meanings.

A. tumor of a gland _____

B. produces fibers _____

C. tissue around cartilage _____

D. nerve glue _____

E. white blood cell _____

F. large phagocytic cell _____

G. bone cell _____

H. a space or cavity within a cell _____

I. a blood clot _____

J. without blood vessels _____

14. For each of the following words, write a sentence that includes the word.

A. histologist

_____

_____

B. ambilateral

_____

_____

C. cohesion

_____

_____

D. pseudoplegia

_____

_____

E. toxin

_____

_____

TESTING COMPREHENSION

1. A tissue that has closely packed cells with very little intercellular material is (a) epithelium, (b) connective, (c) muscle, (d) nerve.

2. The tissue that has macrophages and fibroblasts is (a) epithelium, (b) connective, (c) muscle, (d) nerve.

3. Cells with axons and dendrites are part of what tissue? (a) epithelium, (b) connective, (c) muscle, (d) nerve.

4. The tissue that includes blood and bones is (a) epithelium, (b) connective, (c) muscle, (d) nerve.

5. The tissue that contains the proteins actin and myosin is (a) epithelium, (b) connective, (c) muscle, (d) nerve.

6. The tissue that forms the outer layer of skin is (a) simple squamous epithelium, (b) pseudostratified epithelium, (c) simple columnar epithelium, (d) stratified squamous epithelium.

7. The lining of the urinary bladder is (a) transitional epithelium, (b) pseudostratified epithelium, (c) stratified epithelium, (d) simple epithelium.

8. The tissue that forms the intervertebral disks is (a) epithelium, (b) connective, (c) muscle, (d) nerve.

9. Most of the fetal skeleton is (a) fibrocartilage, (b) elastic cartilage, (c) hyaline cartilage, (d) dense fibrous connective tissue.

10. The tissue that forms tendons and ligament is (a) elastic connective tissue, (b) elastic cartilage, (c) fibrocartilage, (d) dense fibrous connective tissue.

11. Goblet cells are an example of (a) endocrine glands, (b) merocrine glands, (c) apocrine glands, (d) unicellular glands.

12. Ligaments have an abundance of (a) blood vessels, (b) elastic fibers, (c) adipose cells, (d) collagenous fibers.

13. Which of the following is found in both osseous tissue and cartilage? (a) canaliculi, (b) lamellae, (c) lacunae, (d) haversian canals.

14. Involuntary control and cross-striations are characteristic of (a) skeletal muscle, (b) smooth muscle, (c) visceral muscle, (d) cardiac muscle.

15. Membranes that line body cavities that open to the exterior are (a) mucous membranes, (b) synovial membranes, (c) serous membranes, (d) meninges.

53

16. Jackson had an ulcer that eroded the lining of his stomach. The tissue that was damaged was (a) simple squamous epithelium, (b) simple cuboidal epithelium, (c) simple columnar epithelium, (d) transitional epithelium.

17. Lyle damaged the muscle in his shoulder. This muscle (a) was multinucleated, (b) had intercalated disks, (c) was involuntary muscle, (d) had branching fibers.

18. To her dismay, Sonia developed a couple of pimples on her face just before her school's Spring Fling dance. The pimples developed in the openings of the ducts from sebaceous glands. These glands (a) are unicellular glands, (b) are holocrine glands, (c) are similar to sweat glands in their mode of secretion, (d) secrete their product from the cell, but the cell remains intact.

19. Karen was hospitalized with meningitis, an inflammation of the meninges. The meninges are (a) serous membranes, (b) mucous membranes, (c) epithelial membranes, (d) connective tissue membranes.

20. Systemic lupus erythematosus is an autoimmune disease that affects collagen in the body. Collagen is found primarily in (a) epithelial tissue, (b) connective tissue, (c) muscle tissue, (d) nerve tissue.

21. Brenda was diagnosed as having ductile carcinoma of the breast. This indicates a tumor of (a) epithelial tissue, (b) connective tissue, (c) adipose tissue, (d) muscle tissue.

22. Jeremy had a stricture in a blood vessel leading away from the heart This means that the blood vessel (a) had a clot in it, (b) had a breakdown in the vessel wall, (c) had a vacuole in it, (d) had a narrow region in it.

23. The LPN in the extended care facility noticed on Mr. Smith's chart that he was to have ASA ac. These abbreviations mean that he was to have (a) aspirin before meals, (b) aspirin after meals, (c) acetaminophen before meals, (c) acetaminophen after meals.

24. Sharon was diagnosed as having a glioma. Sharon had a tumor in (a) epithelial tissue, (b) connective tissue, (c) muscle tissue, (d) nerve tissue.

25. Sean was diagnosed as having a form of fibroadenia. This disorder involves (a) glands, (b) bones, (c) blood, (d) nerves.

A STEP BEYOND

Go a step beyond the ordinary and learn more about a topic that is related to this chapter but not discussed in detail in the textbook. Select one of the following topics, or one suggested by your instructor, and write a brief paper (250 words minimum), create a poster, or develop a short presentation (approximately 4 to 5 minutes) that focuses on your selection. Suggested topics for this chapter include the following:

1. *Collagen diseases.* Collagen is a major component of connective tissue. For unknown reasons, the body sometimes destroys its own collagen. Select one of the collagen diseases such as rheumatoid arthritis, systemic lupus erythematosus, or scleroderma, and study the pathogenesis, diagnosis, treatment, and prognosis of the disease.
2. *Body weight and fitness.* Maintaining an ideal body weight is a healthy goal. A better indicator of health and fitness is body composition. Learn about the relationships between body weight, body fat, body composition, and fitness.
3. *Tissue typing.* What is tissue typing? What is its purpose? What techniques are used for tissue typing?

Word Scramble

Determine the word that fits each definition, and then write the word in the spaces below the definition, one letter per space. The letters in the boxes form a scrambled word or words. Unscramble the letters to create a word or words that match the final definition in each section.

1. Large phagocytic cell

2. Nerve cell

3. Fatty connective tissue

4. Bone cell

Letters to use for final word: _____

Final definition: Cell eating

_____

5. Study of tissue

6. Abnormal collagen because of vitamin C deficiency

7. Study of the nature of disease

8. Group of cells with similar structure and function

9. Benign tumor of muscle tissue

10. White connective tissue fibers

11. Type of gland that includes salivary and pancreatic glands

Letters to use for final words: _____

Final definition: Chronic autoimmune connective tissue disease

_____

5 Integumentary System

Structure of the Skin

1. The integumentary system includes _____, _____,
_____, and _____.

2. Write the name of the layer or structure that corresponds to each of the descriptions. Select your answers from the following choices.

Dermis	Stratum basale	Stratum granulosum
Epidermis	Stratum corneum	Stratum lucidum
Hypodermis	Stratum germinativum	Stratum spinosum

A. _____ Referred to as the subcutaneous layer

B. _____ Specific layer that contains melanocytes

C. _____ Epidermal layer next to the dermis

D. _____ Consists of stratum basale and stratum spinosum

E. _____ Consists of a papillary layer and a reticular layer

F. _____ Layer immediately above the stratum basale

G. _____ Referred to as superficial fascia

H. _____ Found only in thick skin

I. _____ Keratinization begins in this layer

J. _____ Consists of dead, completely keratinized cells

K. _____ Layer in which hair, nails, and glands are embedded

L. _____ Contains receptors for temperature and touch

M. _____ Contains adipose tissue

N. _____ Actively mitotic layer

O. _____ Has collagen fibers that give strength to the skin

Skin Color

1. What is the name of the dark pigment that is primarily responsible for skin color?

   _____

2. What is the name of the yellow pigment found in the skin?

   _____

3. What accounts for the pink color of the skin?

   _____

4. Explain why a "tan" is temporary.

   _____

   _____

Epidermal Derivatives

1. Write the terms that fit the following descriptive phrases about epidermal derivatives.

   A. _____ Tubular sheath surrounding the hair root

   B. _____ Smooth muscle associated with hair

   C. _____ Epidermal layer that produces hair and nails

   D. _____ Central core of a hair

   E. _____ Crescent-shaped area over the nail matrix

   F. _____ Type of gland generally associated with hair

   G. _____ Glands that produce earwax

   H. _____ Sweat glands that function in temperature regulation

   I. _____ Another name for sweat glands

   J. _____ Enlarged region of hair follicle embedded in dermis

   K. _____ Another name for nail cuticle

   L. _____ Large sweat glands in the axilla

Functions of the Skin

1. Four types of functions of the integument are

   A. _____

   B. _____

   C. _____

   D. _____

2. The protein that is a waterproofing agent in the skin is _____.

3. Bacterial growth on the skin is inhibited by _____.

4. Tissues under the skin are protected from ultraviolet light by _____.

5. Sense receptors for heat, cold, pain, touch, and pressure are located in the _____ of the skin.

6. Describe two mechanisms by which the skin functions in temperature regulation.

   A. blood vessels

   _____

   _____

   B. sweat glands

   _____

   _____

7. How does the skin function in the synthesis of vitamin D?

   _____

   _____

Burns

1. Indicate whether each of the following phrases pertains to first-degree (1), second-degree (2), or third-degree (3) burns. If the phrase pertains to more than one type, indicate this by using all the correct numbers.

   A. _____ requires skin grafts

   B. _____ stratum basale is damaged

   C. _____ heals by regeneration

   D. _____ becomes red

   E. _____ involves subcutaneous tissue

   F. _____ painful

   G. _____ blisters

   H. _____ superficial

   I. _____ may produce scarring

   J. _____ involves the dermis

   K. _____ severe scarring

   L. _____ nerve endings have been destroyed

2. Jack B. Nimble suffered third-degree burns over his anterior trunk and the anterior surface of both arms.

   A. What percentage of his total body surface area had third-degree burns?

   _____

   B. What are the two most important medical challenges presented by this burn?

   _____

LABELING AND COLORING EXERCISES

1. Identify the layers and structures of the skin in the following diagram by placing the correct letter in the space provided by the listed labels. Then select different colors for each structure and use them to color the coding circles and the corresponding structures in the illustration.

_____ Arrector pili muscle ○

_____ Blood vessel ○

_____ Epidermis ○

_____ Hair bulb ○

_____ Sebaceous gland ○

_____ Stratum basale ○

_____ Stratum corneum ○

_____ Sweat gland ○

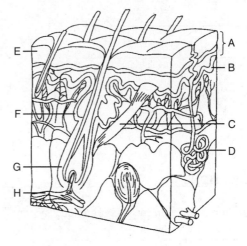

Figure 5-1 Section of the skin.

2. Figure 5-2 shows the structure of hair and hair follicles. Color the shaft brown, the root blue, the sebaceous gland yellow and the arrector pili muscle red. Provide labels for other structures as indicated.

A. _____

B. _____

C. _____

D. _____

E. _____

F. _____

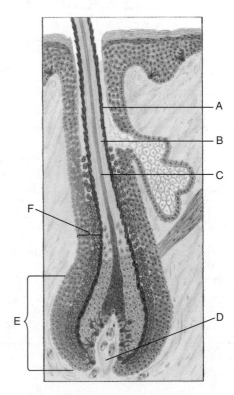

Figure 5-2 Structures of hair and hair follicles.

Chapter **5** **Integumentary System**

3. Figure 5-3 shows the structure of a nail. Color the nail bed red. Label other structures as indicated.

A. _____

B. _____

C. _____

D. _____

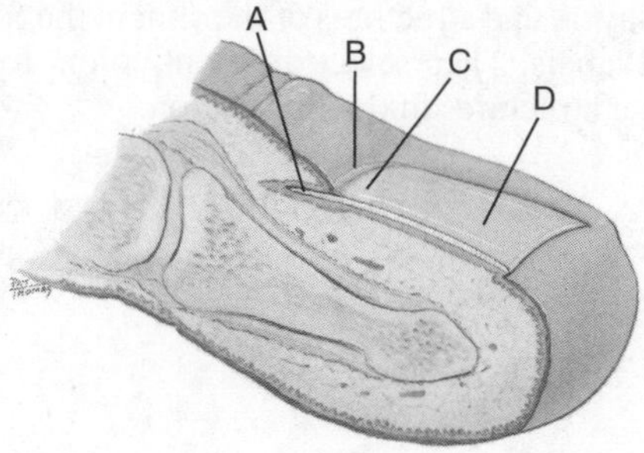

Figure 5-3 Structure of a nail.

REVIEW QUESTIONS

1. What structures make up the integumentary system?

_____

2. What are the epidermis, dermis, and hypodermis?

_____

_____

_____

3. Name the five layers of the epidermis of thick skin and describe the appearance of each layer.

_____

_____

_____

_____

_____

4. What are the features of the two layers of the dermis?

_____

_____

_____

5. Describe two functions of the hypodermis.

_____

_____

6. Discuss two ways in which the integument helps to regulate body temperature.

_____

_____

_____

_____

7. What is the primary factor that determines skin color? Name two additional factors.

_____

_____

8. From what tissue are hair and fingernails derived?

_____

9. Use the following terms in a description of the structure of hair: shaft, root, medulla, cortex, cuticle, hair follicle, hair bulb, papilla, and arrector pili muscle.

_____

_____

_____

10. Use the following terms in a description of the structure of nails: free edge, nail body, nail root, eponychium, nail bed, nail matrix, and lunula.

_____

_____

_____

11. Where are sebaceous glands located? What is their secretory product? What is their function?

_____

_____

12. What is the difference between merocrine and apocrine sudoriferous glands? Where are they located?

_____

_____

13. What are ceruminous glands and where are they located?

_____

_____

14. List four functions of the skin.

_____

_____

15. What are the most serious medical challenges from severe burns?

_____

16. Which two types of burns are painful?

_____

17. Name the skin layers that are damaged in first-, second-, and third-degree burns.

_____

_____

FUNCTIONAL RELATIONSHIPS

It is important to remember that no system in the body works alone. It takes the interaction of all systems to maintain homeostasis. The following exercises reinforce the concept that all systems work together to maintain the health and well-being of other systems and the individual. Match the system on the right with what it provides for the integumentary system on the left.

1. _____ Provides nutrients needed for skin growth

2. _____ Controls cutaneous blood vessel diameter and sweat gland activity

3. _____ Furnishes oxygen and removes carbon dioxide

4. _____ Provides structural support

5. _____ Transports gases and nutrients to skin

6. _____ Protects against skin infections

7. _____ Provides hormones that regulate sebaceous gland activity

8. _____ Provides hormones for maintenance of skin

9. _____ Generates heat

10. _____ Maintains normal fluid composition

A. Skeletal

B. Muscular

C. Nervous

D. Endocrine

E. Cardiovascular

F. Lymphatic

G. Respiratory

H. Digestive

I. Urinary

J. Reproductive

For each of the following systems, write what the integumentary system provides for it.

11. Skeletal _____

12. Cardiovascular _____

13. Muscular _____

14. Reproductive _____

15. Endocrine _____

_____

16. Respiratory _____

17. Nervous _____

18. Lymphatic _____

19. Digestive _____

20. Urinary _____

REPRESENTATIVE DISORDERS

Match the disorder of the integumentary system on the right with its description of the left.

1. _____ Severe inflammation of the dermis and subcutaneous layers		A. Alopecia
2. _____ Allergic transient skin eruptions; hives		B. Cellulitis
		C. Contact dermatitis
3. _____ Elevated pigmented lesion on the skin; mole		D. Eczema
4. _____ Inflammatory skin disease with red, itching, vesicular lesions that may crust over		E. Herpes simplex
		F. Hirsutism
5. _____ Baldness; absence of hair from where it normally grows		G. Nevus
6. _____ Abnormal growth of hair		H. Paronychia
7. _____ Athlete's foot; fungal infection of the skin		I. Ringworm
8. _____ Cold sores, fever blisters		J. Urticaria
9. _____ Inflammation of skin caused by poison ivy and poison oak		
10. _____ Infection involving the folds of soft tissue around the fingernails		

VOCABULARY PRACTICE

1. Match the definitions on the left with the correct term from the column on the right by placing the corresponding number in the space before the definition. Not all terms will be used.

A. _____ Deepest layer of skin damaged in a second-degree burn		1. Alopecia
		2. Dermatitis
B. _____ Baldness		3. Dermis
C. _____ Sunscreen preparation		4. Epidermis
D. _____ A slough produced by a burn or gangrene		5. Eschar
		6. Nevus
E. _____ Severe itching		7. Prophylactic agent
F. _____ A mole		8. Pruritus
G. _____ Inflammation of the skin		9. Therapeutic agent
H. _____ Hives		10. Urticaria

Chapter **5** **Integumentary System**

2. Write the meaning of the following abbreviations:

A. UV _____

B. bx _____

C. FUO _____

D. HSV _____

E. PPD _____

3. Spelling is important in scientific and medical applications because only one or two incorrect letters can change the meaning. Six of the following words from this chapter are misspelled. Place a check mark (√) in the space before the word if it is spelled correctly. Write the correct spelling in the space if it is spelled incorrectly.

A. eczema _____   F. cornium _____

B. impetigo _____   G. lusidum _____

C. carotinization _____   H. arector pili _____

D. sebacious _____   I. eponychium _____

E. subcutaneous _____   J. seruminus _____

4. Write the meaning of the underlined portion of each word on the line following the word.

A. <u>cer</u>uminous _____   F. dermato<u>plasty</u> _____

B. <u>sudor</u>iferous _____   G. <u>xero</u>derma _____

C. <u>ichthy</u>osis _____   H. bacteri<u>cidal</u> _____

D. hyp<u>onych</u>ium _____   I. <u>cyan</u>osis _____

E. gast<u>rectomy</u> _____   J. <u>pedicul</u>osis _____

5. Separate each of the following words into its component parts, give the meaning of each part, and then write the meaning of the entire word.

A. hidradenitis _____

_____

B. mycodermatitis _____

_____

6. From your knowledge of word parts, write words that have the following meanings.

A. An agent that kills bacteria _____

B. Below the skin _____

C. Surgical removal of the appendix _____

D. Condition of producing no sweat _____

E. A fungus condition _____

F. Abnormal thickening of the skin _____

G. Dry skin _____

H. Beneath a nail _____

I. Plastic surgery to remove wrinkles _____

J. Infestation with lice _____

7. For each of the following words, write a sentence that defines the word.

A. melanocyte

_____

B. onychomycosis

_____

C. trichomycosis

_____

D. cyanosis

_____

E. erythema

_____

1. The epidermis is what type of epithelial tissue? (a) simple squamous, (b) transitional, (c) pseudostratified, (d) stratified squamous.

2. In what layer of the epidermis is melanin produced? (a) stratum basale, (b) stratum lucidum, (c) stratum granulosum, (d) stratum corneum.

3. Hair and nails are derived from the (a) stratum corneum, (b) dermis, (c) stratum basale, (d) hypodermis.

4. Which of the following contains the most adipose tissue? (a) stratum basale, (b) hypodermis, (c) stratum corium, (d) papillary layer.

5. The waterproofing feature of the skin comes from the protein (a) collagen, (b) elastin, (c) chondrin, (d) keratin.

6. The papillary layer in the skin is the (a) uppermost layer of the dermis, (b) the uppermost layer of the epidermis, (c) the lower layer of the dermis, (d) the lowest layer of the epidermis.

7. The layer of the skin that is responsible for fingerprints is the (a) stratum corneum, (b) stratum basale, (c) upper layer of the stratum corium, (d) hypodermis.

8. After the birth of her baby, Jenni had white streaks on parts of her abdomen. Her doctor explained that these are called striae and are caused by overstretching the (a) stratum basale, (b) dermis, (c) hypodermis, (d) epidermis.

9. Albinism results from a lack of (a) melanin, (b) carotene, (c) collagen, (d) blood vessels.

10. Dilation of cutaneous blood vessels causes increased blood flow. As a result, the skin becomes (a) pale or white, (b) more yellow because the carotene shows through, (c) red or blushes, (d) darker because melanin is brought to the surface.

11. Julie went to the salon for a new hairstyle. Part of the process involved cutting her hair. The portion that was cut was the (a) bulb, (b) root, (c) follicle, (d) shaft.

12. The central core of hair is the (a) medulla, (b) cortex, (c) shaft, (d) follicle.

13. Which of the following is **not** associated with hair? (a) arrector pili, (b) sebaceous glands, (c) stratum basale, (d) merocrine sweat glands.

14. The crescent-shaped white area opposite the free edge of a nail is the (a) eponychium, (b) cuticle, (c) lunula, (d) nail matrix.

15. Sebaceous glands associated with hair follicles are (a) holocrine glands, (b) apocrine glands, (c) merocrine glands, (d) sudoriferous glands.

16. Which one of the following statements is **not** true about functions of the skin? (a) exposure to ultraviolet light usually increases the activity of melanocytes; (b) secretions of sweat glands help protect against fluid loss; (c) when body temperature increases, the dermal capillaries dilate; (d) vitamin D is produced in the skin in response to ultraviolet light.

17. Which of the following does **not** describe a third-degree burn? (a) hypodermis is involved; (b) blisters form; (c) results in scarring; (d) is a full-thickness burn.

18. Kyle received burns on both of his arms while rescuing his sister from a house fire. Fortunately he recovered without scarring. Approximately how much of his body was burned? (a) 4%; (b) 10%; (c) 18%; (d) 27%.

19. Pimples and blackheads develop in hair follicles, usually on the face. They are associated with (a) ceruminous glands, (b) sebaceous glands, (c) merocrine sweat glands, (d) sudoriferous glands.

20. Sensory receptors in the skin are located in the (a) stratum corneum, (b) stratum spinosum, (c) stratum basale, (d) stratum corium.

21. Sasha went to visit her grandmother in the extended-care facility. She noticed that her grandmother's skin, in addition to being wrinkled, was very thin and almost transparent. She also observed that her grandmother was not able to tolerate environmental temperature changes, especially cold. It seemed that her grandmother was cold all the time, even when others were comfortable. This was probably due to the fact that (a) there was less fat in the hypodermis; (b) her sebaceous glands were secreting less sebum; (c) her stratum corneum was thinner than normal; (d) her melanocytes were producing less melanin.

22. Nate went to a dermatologist because he noticed a growth on his neck. The dermatologist explained that it was an epidermal growth caused by a virus. This growth was probably (a) urticaria, (b) a carcinoma, (c) eczema, (d) a wart.

23. A slough produced by a burn or gangrene is called (a) psoriasis, (b) ecchymosis, (c) eschar, (d) purpura.

24. Severe itching, possibly from an allergic reaction, is called (a) dermatitis, (b) pruritus, (c) petechia, (d) scabies.

25. Cari sustained numerous bruises in an automobile accident. She was told that a bruise is (a) a callus, (b) a pustule, (c) an ecchymosis, (d) a wheal.

A STEP BEYOND

Go a step beyond the ordinary and learn more about a topic that is related to this chapter but not discussed in detail in the textbook. Select one of the following topics, or one suggested by your instructor, and write a brief paper (250 words minimum), create a poster, or develop a short presentation (approximately 4 to 5 minutes) that focuses on your selection. Suggested topics for this chapter include the following:

1. *Sunscreen preparations.* Check the active ingredients in five different brands of sunscreen preparations. Does there seem to be a common ingredient? If so, determine the chemical formula for the ingredient and the properties that make it an effective sunscreen. In other words, how does it work?
2. *Skin cancer.* Summarize the three common types of skin cancer. Include the cells where the cancer originates, risk factors, characteristics, treatment, and prognosis.
3. *Enhancing the integumentary system.* Americans spend millions of dollars each year on products for the integumentary system. Select one product category (shampoo, hand lotion, face cream, liquid makeup, prophylactic acne preparations, etc.) and check the ingredients for five brands in the category you selected. Is there any correlation in the ingredients, either active or inactive? Is there a difference in active ingredients between the inexpensive and expensive products in your category?

Word Scramble

Determine the word that fits each definition, and then write the word in the spaces below the definition, one letter per space. The letters in the boxes form a scrambled word or words. Unscramble the letters to create a word or words that match the final definition in each section.

1. Outermost layer of epidermis

2. Waterproofing protein in epidermis

3. Associated with hair follicles

4. Cuticle

5. Superficial fascia

Letters to use for final words: _____

Final definition: Subject of this chapter

_____

6. Inability to produce melanin

7. Yellowish pigment in skin

8. Earwax

9. Produce perspiration

Letters to use for final words: _____

Final definition: Deepest layer of the epidermis.

_____

6 Skeletal System

Overview of the Skeletal System

1. List five functions of the skeletal system.

   A. _____

   B. _____

   C. _____

   D. _____

   E. _____

2. Place an "S" before each phrase that pertains to spongy bone and a "C" before each phrase that pertains to compact bone.

   A. _____ Closely packed osteons

   B. _____ Contains red bone marrow

   C. _____ Trabeculae

   D. _____ Canaliculi radiate from lacunae to osteonic canal

   E. _____ Contains irregular spaces

3. Place an "L" before each phrase that pertains to long bones, an "S" before each phrase that pertains to short bones, and an "F" before each phrase that pertains to flat bones.

   A. _____ Has a diploe of spongy bone

   B. _____ Vertical dimension longer than the horizontal dimension

   C. _____ Roughly cube-shaped

   D. _____ Primarily spongy bone covered with a thin layer of compact bone

   E. _____ Bones in the wrist and ankle

   F. _____ Bones in the thigh and arm

   G. _____ Spongy bone between two layers of compact bone

4. Write the terms that fit the following descriptive phrase about the features of long bone.

A. _____ Tubular shaft of a long bone

B. _____ Expanded ends of long bone

C. _____ Outer covering of a long bone

D. _____ Hollow region in the shaft

E. _____ Hyaline cartilage that covers the ends of the bone

F. _____ Connective tissue membrane that lines the shaft

5. Write the terms that fit the following descriptive phrases about bone markings.

A. _____ Smooth, rounded articular surface

B. _____ Opening through a bone

C. _____ Smooth shallow depression

D. _____ Cavity or hollow space in a bone

E. _____ Smooth, flat articular surface

F. _____ Large, blunt projections found on the femur

6. Write the terms that fit the following descriptive phrases about bone development and growth.

A. _____ Process of bone formation

B. _____ Cells that deposit bone matrix; bone-forming cells

C. _____ Mature bone cells located in lacunae

D. _____ Cells that destroy bone by removing bone matrix

E. _____ Type of ossification in most flat bones of the skull

F. _____ Bone development in which hyaline cartilage models are replaced by bone

G. _____ Region where long bones increase in length

H. _____ Cells in the periosteum that are responsible for increase in bone diameter

I. _____ Cells that hollow out the medullary cavity

J. _____ Type of ossification in most long bones of the body

7. A. _____ Number of named bones in the complete skeleton

B. _____ Number of named bones in the axial skeleton

C. _____ Number of named bones in the appendicular skeleton

Bones of the Axial Skeleton

1. Name the bones that form the cranium and indicate how many there are of each one.

_____

_____

_____

2. Name the bones that form the face and indicate how many there are of each one.

_____

_____

_____

3. For each of the following, name the bone of the skull that has the given feature:

A. _____ Foramen magnum   E. _____ Optic foramen

B. _____ Auditory meatus   F. _____ Cribriform plate

C. _____ Supraorbital foramen   G. _____ Sella turcica

D. _____ Mastoid process   H. _____ Ramus

4. What is the name of the U-shaped bone in the neck? _____

5. Write the terms that fit the following descriptive phrases about the axial skeleton.

A. _____ First cervical vertebra

B. _____ Vertebrae that articulate with ribs

C. _____ Weight-bearing portion of a vertebra

D. _____ Superior portion of the breastbone

E. _____ Second cervical vertebra

F. _____ Type of vertebrae in the neck

G. _____ Vertebrae with heavy bodies and blunt processes

H. _____ Another name for the breastbone

I. _____ Cartilaginous pads between the vertebrae

6. State the number for each of the following:

A. _____ True ribs   C. _____ Cervical vertebrae

B. _____ Lumbar vertebrae   D. _____ Vertebrosternal ribs

Chapter **6** **Skeletal System**

E. _____ False ribs   G. _____ Thoracic vertebrae

F. _____ Vertebral ribs   H. _____ Vertebrochondral ribs

Bones of the Appendicular Skeleton

1. Identify the bone or feature of the pectoral girdle and upper extremity that best fists each description given below.

A. _____ Anterior bone of the pectoral girdle

B. _____ Posterior bone of the pectoral girdle

C. _____ Bone that has an acromion and spine

D. _____ Large bone in the arm

E. _____ Bone on the lateral side of the forearm

F. _____ Bone on the medial side of the forearm

G. _____ Wrist bones

H. _____ Bones that form the palm of the hand

I. _____ Bones that form the fingers and toes

J. _____ Bone that articulates with the trochlea of humerus

K. _____ Bone that articulates with capitulum of humerus

L. _____ Projection on proximal end of ulna

2. Identify the bone or feature of the pelvic girdle and lower extremity that best fits each description given below.

A. _____ Three bones that fuse to form the os coxa

   _____

   _____

B. _____ Depression in the os coxa for the femoral head

C. _____ Portion of femur that articulates with tibia

D. _____ Bone on the medial side of the leg

E. _____ Bone on the lateral side of the leg

F. _____ Tarsal that forms the heel

G. _____ Tarsal that articulates with the tibia

H. _____ Bone in tendon anterior to femur and tibia

I. _____ Bone of axial skeleton articulating with os coxa

J. _____ Bone that has greater and lesser trochanters

3. Compare the pelvis in the male and female by completing the following table.

Feature	Male	Female
Pubic arch		
Pelvic inlet		
Pelvic cavity		

4. The portion of the pelvis between the flared wings of the ilium bones is called the _____ pelvis.

The portion inferior to the pelvic brim is the _____ pelvis.

Fractures and Fracture Repair

1. Identify the following fractures by writing the name of the fracture on the line preceding the description.

A. _____ Broken bone protrudes through the skin

B. _____ Bone is crushed into multiple small pieces

C. _____ Break is at right angles to the bone's long axis

D. _____ Broken ends of the bone are not correctly aligned

E. _____ Bone is broken by twisting

2. Six-year-old Johnny Showman fell on his shoulder while at the playground. Radiographs showed that the right clavicle was connected on one surface of the bone but that the other surface was broken.

A. Is this fracture open or closed?

B. Is this fracture complete or incomplete?

C. Arrange the events of fracture repair for Johnny's clavicle in the correct sequence by placing numbers 1 through 5 on the lines with 1 being the first event and 5 being the final event.

_____ Bony callus

_____ Fracture hematoma

_____ Remodeling

_____ Procallus

_____ Fibrocartilaginous callus

Articulations

1. Indicate whether each of the following pertains to synarthroses, amphiarthroses, or diarthroses by writing the correct letter in the space provided before each descriptive phrase. S= synarthroses, A = amphiarthroses, D = diarthroses.

A. _____ Sutures   F. _____ Ball and socket

B. _____ Slightly movable   G. _____ Ribs to sternum

C. _____ Meniscus   H. _____ May have bursae

D. _____ Immovable   I. _____ Joint capsule

E. _____ Elbow and knee   J. _____ Symphysis pubis

LABELING AND COLORING EXERCISES

Identify the bones and selected features of the skull in the following diagram by placing the correct letter in the space provided by the listed labels. Then select a different color for each bone and use it to color the coding circles and the corresponding bone in the illustration.

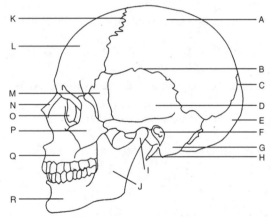

Figure 6-1 Skull, lateral view.

_____ Frontal ○   _____ Parietal ○   _____ Lambdoidal suture ○

_____ Lacrimal ○   _____ Sphenoid ○   _____ Mandibular condyle ○

_____ Mandible ○   _____ Temporal ○   _____ Mastoid process ○

_____ Maxilla ○   _____ Zygomatic ○   _____ Ramus ○

_____ Nasal ○   _____ Auditory meatus ○   _____ Squamosal suture ○

_____ Occipital ○   _____ Coronal suture ○   _____ Styloid process ○

2. Label the general features of vertebrae as indicated in Figure 6-2.

A. _____

B. _____

C. _____

D. _____

E. _____

F. _____

G. _____

H. _____

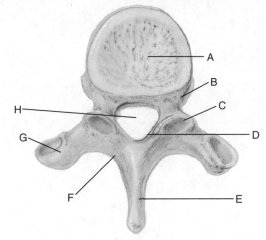

Figure 6-2 General features of vertebrae.

3. Label the features of the sternum as indicated in Figure 6-3. Color the vertebrosternal ribs red, the vertebrochondral ribs blue, and the vertebral ribs yellow.

A. _____

B. _____

C. _____

D. _____

E. _____

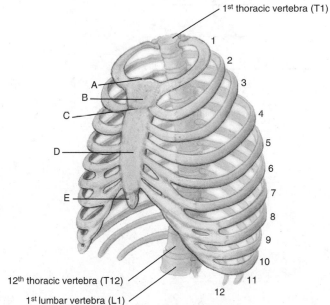

Figure 6-3 Thoracic cage.

4. Identify the bones indicated on the anterior view of the skeleton shown in Figure 6-4, and then color the axial skeleton red and the appendicular skeleton blue.

A. _____

B. _____

C. _____

D. _____

E. _____

F. _____

G. _____

H. _____

I. _____

J. _____

K. _____

L. _____

M. _____

N. _____

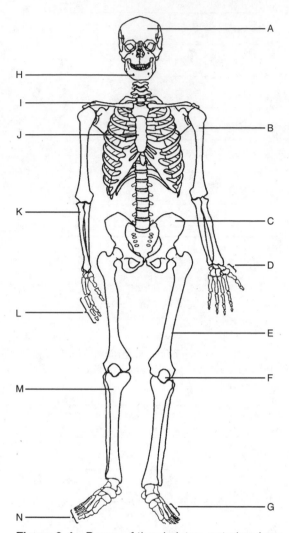

Figure 6-4 Bones of the skeleton, anterior view.

5. Identify the bones indicated on the posterior view of the skeleton shown in Figure 6-5, and then color the axial skeleton red and the appendicular skeleton blue.

A. _____

B. _____

C. _____

D. _____

E. _____

F. _____

G. _____

H. _____

I. _____

J. _____

K. _____

L. _____

M. _____

N. _____

O. _____

P. _____

Q. _____

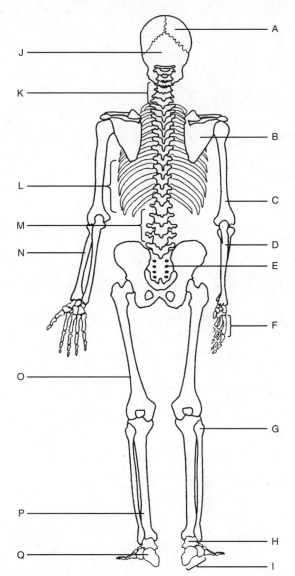

Figure 6-5 Bones of the skeleton, posterior view.

6. Identify the components of a synovial joint as indicated in Figure 6-6.

A. _____

B. _____

C. _____

D. _____

E. _____

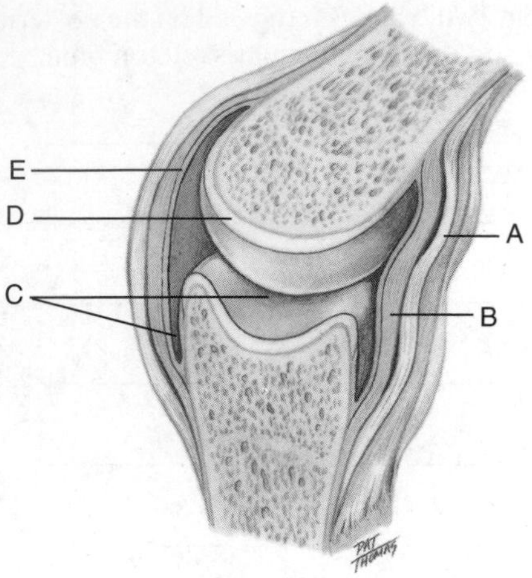

Figure 6-6 Components of a synovial joint.

7. Identify each type of fracture shown in Figure 6-7.

A. _____

B. _____

C. _____

D. _____

E. _____

F. _____

G. _____

H. _____

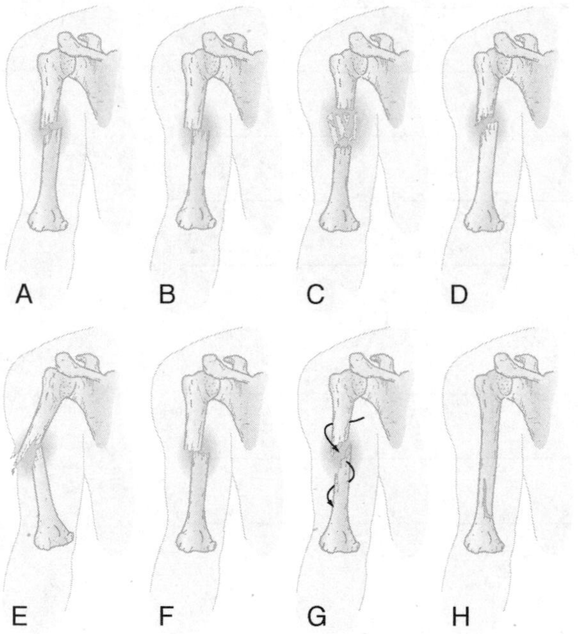

Figure 6-7 Types of fractures.

REVIEW QUESTIONS

1. List five functions of the skeletal system.

_____

_____

_____

2. What is the difference between compact bone and spongy bone? Where is each one located?

_____

_____

_____

_____

_____

3. Give examples of long bones, short bones, flat bones, and irregular bones.

_____

_____

_____

_____

4. Draw and label the general features of a typical long bone.

5. What are osteoblasts, osteoclasts, and osteocytes?

_____

_____

_____

6. How does intramembranous ossification differ from endochondral ossification?

_____

_____

_____

7. Where in the bone do bones increase in length? How do they increase in diameter?

_____

_____

_____

_____

8. How many bones are in the axial skeleton? Appendicular skeleton?

_____

9. Name the eight bones of the cranium and indicate how many there are of each.

_____

_____

10. Name the 14 bones of the face and indicate how many there are of each.

_____

_____

_____

11. What are auditory ossicles, and where are they located?

_____

_____

12. What is unique about the hyoid bone?

_____

_____

13. What are the four curvatures of the vertebral column, and when do they develop? What is their purpose?

_____

_____

_____

_____

14. What features are common to most vertebrae?

_____

_____

_____

15. Identify at least two characteristics that are unique to cervical vertebrae, to thoracic vertebrae, and to lumbar vertebrae. How many of each type of vertebrae are there?

_____

_____

_____

_____

16. Where are the sacrum and coccyx located? What are their features?

_____

_____

_____

17. What are the three parts of the sternum?

_____

18. What is the difference between vertebral ribs, vertebrosternal ribs, and vertebrochondral ribs?

_____

_____

_____

19. What bones are in the pectoral girdle?

_____

20. Name the bones of the upper extremity and tell where they are located.

_____

_____

_____

_____

21. What three bones fuse to form an os coxa?

_____

22. Define or describe each of the following:

A. symphysis pubis _____

B. acetabulum _____

C. iliosacral joint _____

D. obturator foramen _____

E. iliac crest _____

F. greater sciatic notch _____

G. ischial tuberosity _____

23. What is the difference between the false pelvis and the true pelvis?

_____

_____

24. Name the bones of the lower extremity and tell where they are located.

_____

_____

_____

_____

_____

_____

_____

25. What is the difference between open and closed fractures? Transverse and spiral fractures?

_____

_____

_____

26. List the five steps of fracture repair in the sequence in which they occur.

_____

_____

_____

27. What are three types of joints based on the amount of movement they permit? Give at least one example of each type.

_____

_____

_____

28. List five structural features present in all synovial joints.

_____

_____

29. What are menisci and bursae? What is their purpose?

_____

_____

30. Name six different types of freely movable joints.

_____

_____

FUNCTIONAL RELATIONSHIPS

It is important to remember that no system in the body works alone. It takes the interaction of all systems to maintain homeostasis. The following exercises reinforce the concept that all systems work together to maintain the health and well-being of other systems and the individual. Match the system on the right with what it provides for the skeletal system on the left. Use the functional relationships page in your concepts textbook as a resource.

1. _____ Stabilizes position of bones

2. _____ Assists in repair of bone tissue following trauma

3. _____ Absorbs nutrients for bone growth

4. _____ Produces hormones that influence bone growth

5. _____ Synthesis of vitamin D for bone growth

6. _____ Supplies oxygen for bone metabolism

7. _____ Interprets impulses relating to pain in bones

8. _____ Provides hormones that regulate calcium uptake in bones

9. _____ Removes metabolic wastes from bones

10. _____ Conserves calcium and phosphate ions for bones

A. Muscular
B. Nervous
C. Endocrine
D. Cardiovascular
E. Integumentary
F. Lymphatic
G. Respiratory
H. Digestive
I. Urinary
J. Reproductive

For each of the following systems, write what the skeletal system provides for it.

11. Cardiovascular _____

12. Muscular _____

13. Reproductive _____

14. Endocrine _____

15. Respiratory _____

16. Nervous _____

17. Lymphatic _____

18. Digestive _____

19. Urinary _____

20. Integumentary _____

REPRESENTATIVE DISORDERS

Match the disorder of the skeletal system on the right with its description of the left.

1. _____ Incomplete dislocation of a joint

2. _____ Inflammation of a joint

3. _____ Uric acid crystals develop within a joint

4. _____ Softening of bone that occurs in childhood because of inadequate calcium and phosphorus

5. _____ Malignant tumor derived from bone

6. _____ Displacement of a bone from its joint

7. _____ Inflammation of bone marrow

8. _____ Overstretching of a muscle over a joint

9. _____ Decrease in bone density or mass

10. _____ Twisting of a joint with injury to ligaments, tendons, muscles, and blood vessels

A. Arthritis
B. Dislocation
C. Gout
D. Osteomyelitis
E. Osteoporosis
F. Osteosarcoma
G. Rickets
H. Sprain
I. Strain
J. Subluxation

VOCABULARY PRACTICE

Match the definitions on the left with the correct term from the column on the right by placing the corresponding letter in the space before the definition. Not all terms will be used.

1. _____ Shaft of a long bone

2. _____ Uric acid crystals develop within a joint causing acute inflammation

3. _____ Bone-forming cell

4. _____ Congenital deformity of the foot; clubfoot

5. _____ Ibuprofen

6. _____ Displacement of a bone from its joint with tearing of the articular cartilage

7. _____ Inflammation of a joint

8. _____ Twisting of a joint with injury to ligaments, tendons, muscles, blood vessels, nerves

9. _____ Acetaminophen

10. _____ Slightly movable joint

A. Amphiarthrosis
B. Arthritis
C. Diaphysis
D. Dislocation
E. Gout
F. NSAID (nonsteroidal anti-inflammatory drug)
G. Osteoblast
H. Osteoclast
I. Sprain
J. Synarthrosis
K. Talipes
L. Tylenol

11. Write the meaning of the following abbreviations.

A. ACL _____   F. EMG _____

B. CTS _____   G. NSAID _____

C. ROM _____   H. TMJ _____

D. fx _____   I. SI _____

E. THR _____   J. RA _____

12. Spelling is important in scientific and medical applications because only one or two incorrect letters can change the meaning. All of the following words from this chapter are misspelled. Write the correct spelling in the space provided following the word.

A. symarthrosis _____

B. ileum _____

C. carpel _____

D. fibia _____

E. falanges _____

13. Write the meaning of the underlined portion of each word on the line following the word.

A. kyphosis _____   F. bursa _____

B. hematopoiesis _____   G. cribriform _____

C. spondylosis _____   H. synarthroses _____

D. osteoarthritis _____   I. ethmoid _____

E. osteomyelitis _____   J. chondrocostal _____

14. Using the following word parts, write words that fit the given definitions.

| -algia | chondr- | -ectomy | -pathy |
| arthr- | cost- | osteo- | phalang- |

A. Excision of a finger or toe _____

B. Pain in the ribs _____

C. Disease of cartilage _____

D. Surgical removal of a joint _____

E. Any disease of both bones and joints _____

15. Separate each of the following words into its component parts, give the meaning of each part, and then write the meaning of the entire word.

A. osteoplasty

_____

_____

_____

B. ankylosis

_____

_____

_____

16. Match the clinical terms on the right with their descriptions on the left.

A. _____ Visual examination of the inside of a joint

B. _____ Physician who specializes in the treatment of bone and joint diseases

C. _____ Abnormal protrusion of an intervertebral disk into the neural canal

D. _____ Abnormal swelling of the joint between the big toe and first metatarsal

E. _____ A physician who specializes in the treatment of joint diseases

F. _____ Degenerative joint disease

G. _____ Surgical puncture to remove fluid from a joint cavity

H. _____ Bony growth arising from the surface of a bone

I. _____ Developmental anomaly in which the vertebral laminae do not close around the spinal cord

J. _____ Uses physical means to manipulate the spinal column; not a physician

1. Arthrocenteses
2. Arthroscopy
3. Bunion
4. Chiropractor
5. Exostosis
6. Herniated disk
7. Orthopedist
8. Osteoarthritis
9. Rheumatologist
10. Spina bifida

TESTING COMPREHENSION

Multiple choice: Select the best response.

1. The matrix of bone tissue is deposited in concentric rings called (a) osteons, (b) lamellae, (c) lacunae, (d) canaliculi.

2. Bone cells are located in spaces called (a) osteons, (b) lamellae, (c) lacunae, (d) canaliculi.

3. The plates of bone tissue in cancellous bone are called (a) lamellae, (b) lacunae, (c) canaliculi, (d) trabeculae.

4. Intramembranous ossification occurs in the (a) frontal bone, (b) vertebrae, (c) femur, (d) phalanges.

5. Hyaline cartilage is found in the (a) epiphyseal plate, (b) fontanels, (c) endosteum, (d) diploe.

6. Appositional growth is accomplished by (a) osteoblasts and osteoclasts, (b) osteocytes and osteoclasts, (c) osteoblasts and osteocytes, (d) osteocytes and chondrocytes.

7. Wormian bones are bones that grow in (a) tendons, (b) the wrist, (c) the vertebral column, (d) sutures of the skull.

8. The skull contains (a) eight bones, (b) 28 bones, (c) 14 bones, (d) 22 bones.

9. Which of the following are bones of the axial skeleton? (a) clavicle and scapula, (b) ilium and ischium, (c) ribs and sternum, (d) carpals and tarsals.

10. Bones of the cranium include the (a) temporal and palatine, (b) sphenoid and ethmoid, (c) ethmoid and zygomatic, (d) occipital and lacrimal.

11. The bone that has a mastoid process is the (a) temporal, (b) parietal, (c) occipital, (d) mandible.

12. The optic nerve passes through the optic foramen in the (a) sphenoid bone, (b) ethmoid bone, (c) frontal bone, (d) zygomatic bone.

13. The vertebral column contains (a) 22 vertebrae; (b) 30 vertebrae; (c) 12 vertebrae; (d) 26 vertebrae.

14. A feature that distinguishes cervical vertebrae from other types is (a) spinous processes, (b) transverse foramina, (c) vertebral foramina, (d) sacral foramina.

15. The true ribs are also called (a) vertebral ribs, (b) floating ribs, (c) vertebrochondral ribs, (d) vertebrosternal ribs.

16. In anatomic position, the olecranon fossa is (a) on the posterior surface of the proximal ulna, (b) on the anterior surface of the distal humerus, (c) on the posterior surface of the distal humerus, (d) on the anterior surface of the proximal ulna.

17. The trochlear notch is on the (a) humerus, (b) ulna, (c) radius, (d) scapula.

18. When Jenny fractured a metacarpal bone, she fractured a bone in her (a) forearm, (b) wrist, (c) hand, (d) fingers.

19. The portion of the os coxa that articulates with the sacrum is the (a) ilium, (b) ischium, (c) pubis, (d) acetabulum.

20. The largest tarsal bone is the (a) talus, (b) calcaneus, (c) cuboid, (d) navicular.

21. The following are events in the repair of a fracture: (1) bony callus, (2) procallus, (3) remodeling, (4) fracture hematoma, (5) fibrocartilaginous callus. Arrange these events in the correct sequence. (a) 4, 2, 5, 1, 3; (b) 2, 5, 4, 1, 3; (c) 5, 2, 4, 3, 1; (d) 1, 2, 4, 5, 3.

22. An amphiarthrosis is (a) a ball-and-socket joint, (b) an immovable joint, (c) a hinge joint, (d) an intervertebral joint.

23. Bursae are found in some (a) sutures, (b) symphysis joints, (c) diarthrotic joints, (d) synarthrotic joints.

24. The TMJ involves the (a) talus and medial malleolus, (b) temporal bone and mandible, (c) temporal bone and maxillae, (d) tibia and metatarsals.

25. Justin was injured in a football game. Tests showed that he had a torn meniscus. What joint was most likely involved? (a) knee, (b) shoulder, (c) ankle, (d) elbow.

A STEP BEYOND

Go a step beyond the ordinary and learn more about a topic that is related to this chapter but not discussed in detail in the textbook. Select one of the following topics, or one suggested by your instructor, and write a brief paper (250 words minimum), create a poster, or develop a short presentation (approximately 4 to 5 minutes) that focuses on your selection. Suggested topics for this chapter include the following:

1. *Osteoporosis*. What is osteoporosis? Learn about this condition. Include a description of the disease, risk factors, screening techniques, and prevention.
2. *Rickets*. What is rickets? What causes it? What are the characteristics? Learn about this condition and report your findings.
3. *Arthritis*. What is the difference between osteoarthritis and rheumatoid arthritis? Describe each condition. Include the pathogenesis, treatment, and prognosis.

FUN & GAMES

Word Scramble

Determine the word that fits each definition, and then write the word in the spaces below the definition, one letter per space. The letters in the boxes form a scrambled word or words. Unscramble the letters to create a word or words that match the final definition in each section.

1. Middle layer of flat bones

2. Type of ossification in flat bones of the skull

3. Occurs in red bone marrow

Letters to use for final word: _____

Final definition: Bone-forming cells

_____

4. Growth region of a long bone

5. A smooth, shallow depression

6. A tubelike passageway in bone

7. Cancellous bone

8. Tough fibrous covering around bone

9. Bones that grow in tendons

Letters to use for final word: _____

Final definition: Large opening in the occipital bone

_____

Muscular System

LEARNING EXERCISES

Characteristics and Functions of the Muscular System

1. Match the correct type of muscle tissue with each descriptive word or phrase.

A. _____ Striated and involuntary   Skeletal

B. _____ Spindle-shaped fibers   Visceral

C. _____ Multinucleated and cylindrical   Cardiac

D. _____ Found in blood vessels

E. _____ Found in the heart

2. List four characteristics of muscle tissue that relate to its functions.

_____

_____

_____

_____

3. Three functions of muscle contraction are:

_____

_____

_____

Structure of Skeletal Muscle

1. Write the terms that fit the following descriptive phrases in the space provided.

A. _____ More movable attachment of a muscle

B. _____ Covering around an individual muscle fiber

C. _____ Protein in thick myofilaments

D. _____ Bundle of fibers surrounded by perimysium

E. _____ Less movable attachment of a muscle

F. _____ Broad, flat sheet of tendon

G. _____ Cell membrane of a muscle cell

89

H. _____ Protein in thin myofilaments

I. _____ Unit of muscle between Z lines

J. _____ Type of myofilament in the I band

2. Muscle fibers must be stimulated before they can contract; therefore they have an abundant _____.
   The blood supply delivers _____ and _____ for contraction.

Contraction of Skeletal Muscle

1. Arrange the following events of muscle contraction in the correct sequence by writing a number 1 before the first event, number 2 before the second event, and so forth until the eight events have been numbered correctly.

_____ Energized myosin heads attach to actin

_____ Acetylcholine is released into synaptic cleft

_____ Power stroke pulls actin toward the center of the A band

_____ Calcium reacts with troponin and exposes binding sites on actin

_____ Acetylcholine reacts with receptors on sarcolemma

_____ Nerve impulse reaches axon terminal

_____ Calcium ions are released from the sarcoplasmic reticulum

_____ Impulse travels into the T tubules

2. Write the terms that match the statements in the spaces provided.

A. _____ Minimum stimulus that causes contraction

B. _____ Principle by which muscle fibers contract

C. _____ Stimulus insufficient to cause contraction

D. _____ Single neuron and muscle fibers it stimulates

E. _____ Increases contraction strength in a muscle

F. _____ Sustained contraction due to rapid stimuli

G. _____ Staircase effect due to a series of stimuli

H. _____ Continued state of partial muscle contraction

I. _____ Muscle contraction with constant tension

J. _____ Muscle contraction with changing tension

3. Write the terms that match the statements in the spaces provided.

A. _____   Immediate source of energy for contraction

B. _____   Stored in muscle to regenerate adenosine triphosphate (ATP)

C. _____   Molecule that stores oxygen in muscle

D. _____   Acid that accumulates with lack of oxygen

E. _____   Products of aerobic breakdown of pyruvic acid

4. The muscle that has a primary role in providing a movement is called the _____. Muscles that assist this muscle are called _____ and muscles that oppose the movement are called _____.

5. Match the type of muscle movement with the description. Not all responses will be used.

A. _____ Extension of foot to stand on tiptoes

B. _____ Movement of arm toward the midline

C. _____ Straightening the arm at the elbow

D. _____ Turning the palm of the hand forward

E. _____ Turning the head from side to side

F. _____ Moving elbow to put hand on shoulder

G. _____ Turning the sole of foot inward

H. _____ Spreading the fingers apart

I. _____ Tilting the head backward

J. _____ Drawing circles on a chalkboard

1. flexion
2. extension
3. hypertension
4. dorsiflexion
5. plantar flexion
6. abduction
7. adduction
8. rotation
9. supination
10. pronation
11. circumduction
12. inversion
13. eversion

Skeletal Muscle Groups

1. Write the type of muscle feature that is indicated by each of the following muscle names: size, shape, direction of fibers, location, number of origins, origin or insertion, or action.

A. _____   Adductor

B. _____   Rectus

C. _____   Maximus

D. _____   Gluteus

E. _____   Deltoid

F. _____   Biceps

G. _____ Brachioradialis

H. _____ Pectoralis

2. Write the name of the muscle that matches each action.

A. _____ Raises the eyebrows

B. _____ Closes and puckers the lips

C. _____ Raises the mandible in chewing (2)

_____

D. _____ Closes the eye in squinting

E. _____ Flexes neck so the chin drops

F. _____ Primary muscle in inspiration

G. _____ Anterior muscle that adducts and flexes arm

H. _____ Posterior muscle that adducts arm

I. _____ Abducts the arm

J. _____ Extends the forearm

K. _____ Has two heads and flexes forearm

L. _____ Inserts on ulna and flexes forearm

M. _____ Inserts on femur; flexes thigh

N. _____ Synergist of iliopsoas

O. _____ Antagonist of iliopsoas

P. _____ Group that adducts thigh

Q. _____ Group that extends the leg

R. _____ Muscles that flex the leg (3)

_____

_____

S. _____ Muscles that plantar flex the foot (2)

_____

T. _____ Antagonist of the gastrocnemius

LABELING AND COLORING EXERCISES

1. Figure 7-1 illustrates a sarcomere of a skeletal muscle myofibril. Color the actin filaments red and the myosin filaments blue. Label the bands and lines as indicated.

A. _____

B. _____

C. _____

D. _____

E. _____

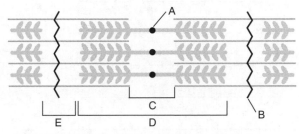

Figure 7-1 Skeletal muscle myofibril.

2. Figure 7-2 illustrates a neuromuscular junction. Color the nerve fiber yellow, the synaptic vesicles blue, and the muscle fiber red. Identify components as indicated.

A. _____

B. _____

C. _____

D. _____

E. _____

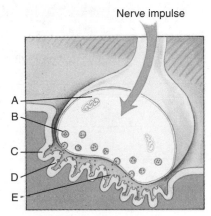

Figure 7-2 Neuromuscular junction.

3. Identify the muscles indicated on Figure 7-3.

A. _____

B. _____

C. _____

D. _____

E. _____

F. _____

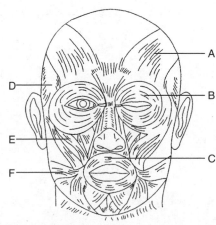

Figure 7-3 Muscles of the head and neck.

Chapter **7 Muscular System**

4. Identify the muscles indicated in Figure 7-4.

A. _____

B. _____

C. _____

D. _____

E. _____

F. _____

G. _____

H. _____

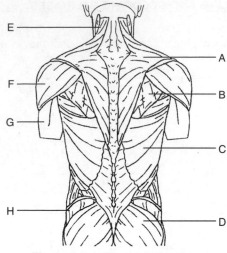

Figure 7-4   Posterior muscles.

5. Identify the muscles indicated on Figure 7-5.

A. _____

B. _____

C. _____

D. _____

E. _____

F. _____

G. _____

H. _____

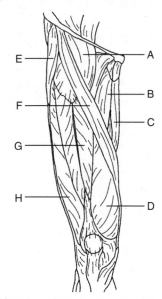

Figure 7-5   Muscles of the lower extremity, anterior view.

6. Identify the muscles indicated on Figure 7-6.

A. _____

B. _____

C. _____

D. _____

E. _____

F. _____

G. _____

H. _____

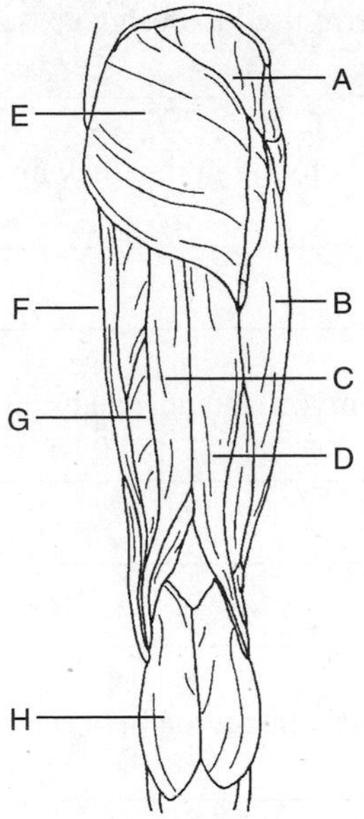

Figure 7-6   Muscles of the lower extremity, posterior view.

REVIEW QUESTIONS

1. How does the appearance of skeletal muscle differ from that of visceral muscle?

   _____

   _____

   _____

2. What are four characteristics of muscle tissue?

   _____

   _____

   _____

   _____

3. Skeletal muscles produce movement. What are two other functions of skeletal muscle tissue?

   _____

   _____

4. What are the endomysium, epimysium, and perimysium?

   _____

   _____

   _____

5. What is the term used to designate the more movable attachment of a muscle?

_____

6. What protein is found in the thick myofilaments? What protein is found in the thin myofilaments?

_____

_____

7. What type of myofilaments makes up the (a) A band, (b) I band, (c) H band?

_____

_____

_____

8. What designates the region between two successive Z lines?

_____

_____

9. Why does skeletal muscle need an abundant blood and nerve supply?

_____

_____

_____

10. What is the neurotransmitter that is released at the neuromuscular junction to stimulate the muscle fiber?

_____

11. What changes occur in the configuration of actin that allow cross-bridges to form between the actin and myosin? What ion is responsible for the changes?

_____

_____

_____

12. Write a sentence that defines the all-or-none principle.

_____

_____

13. What is a motor unit?

_____

14. What is the difference between multiple motor unit summation and multiple wave summation?

_____

_____

_____

15. What type of muscle contraction is responsible for producing movement?

_____

16. What are the immediate, intermediate, and long-term sources of energy for muscle contraction?

_____

_____

_____

17. What organic molecule accumulates when oxygen debt occurs?

_____

18. How do synergists and antagonists relate to the prime mover in a muscle action?

_____

_____

19. What is the opposite of (a) flexion, (b) abduction, (c) pronation, (d) dorsiflexion?

_____

_____

_____

20. Identify the (a) two circular muscles of the face, (b) muscle that elevates the corner of the mouth to form a smile, (c) two muscles that close the jaw when chewing, (d) muscle in the neck that is antagonistic to the sternocleidomastoid.

_____

_____

_____

_____

21. Name the four muscles that constitute the anterolateral abdominal wall.

_____

_____

_____

_____

22. What muscle is antagonistic to the external intercostal muscles?

_____

97

23. Name two muscles that move the shoulder.

_____

_____

24. What is the function of the (a) deltoid, (b) pectoralis major, (c) latissimus dorsi?

_____

_____

_____

25. Name (a) two muscles that are synergists of the biceps brachii and (b) one muscle that is an antagonist of the biceps brachii.

_____

_____

_____

26. Name the muscle that is (a) a synergist of the iliopsoas and (b) an antagonist of the iliopsoas.

_____

_____

27. Identify four muscles that adduct the thigh.

_____

_____

_____

_____

28. What three muscles make up the hamstrings? What is their function?

_____

_____

_____

29. What four muscles make up the quadriceps femoris? What is their function?

_____

_____

_____

_____

30. What muscle that moves the leg is the longest muscle in the body?

_____

31. What two muscle tendons join to form the Achilles tendon?

_____

_____

32. What muscle is in the anterior compartment of the leg and dorsiflexes the foot?

_____

FUNCTIONAL RELATIONSHIPS

It is important to remember that no system in the body works alone. It takes the interaction of all systems to maintain homeostasis. The following exercises reinforce the concept that all systems work together to maintain the health and well-being of other systems and the individual.

Match the system on the right with what it provides for the muscular system on the left. Use the functional relationships page in your concepts textbook as a resource.

1. _____ Produces hormones that affect muscle development and size

2. _____ Provides a barrier against harmful substances

3. _____ Eliminates metabolic waste from muscle contraction

4. _____ Provides attachment sites for muscles

5. _____ Absorbs nutrients for muscle growth and maintenance

6. _____ Coordinates muscle contraction

7. _____ Influences muscle metabolism, mass, and strength

8. _____ Delivers oxygen and nutrients to muscles tissue and removes wastes

9. _____ Maintains interstitial fluid balance in muscle tissue; assists in defense against disease

10. _____ Supplies oxygen for muscle contraction

A. Cardiovascular
B. Digestive
C. Endocrine
D. Integumentary
E. Lymphatic
F. Nervous
G. Reproductive
H. Respiratory
I. Skeletal
J. Urinary

For each of the following systems, write what the muscular system provides for it.

11. Cardiovascular _____

12. Skeletal _____

13. Reproductive _____

14. Endocrine _____

15. Respiratory _____

16. Nervous _____

17. Lymphatic _____

18. Digestive _____

19. Urinary _____

20. Integumentary _____

REPRESENTATIVE DISORDERS

Match the disorder of the skeletal system on the right with its description of the left.

1. _____ An acute contagious, viral disease that causes paralysis

2. _____ Inflammation of muscle tissue

3. _____ Severe form of blood poisoning that inhibits impulses at neuromuscular junctions

4. _____ Muscle remains intact but here is bleeding into surrounding tissue

5. _____ Progressive wasting and weakening of muscles

6. _____ Autoimmune disease characterized by weakness of skeletal muscles

A. Botulism
B. Muscular bruises
C. Muscular dystrophy
D. Myasthenia gravis
E. Myositis
F. Polio

VOCABULARY PRACTICE

Match the definitions on the left with the correct clinical term from the column on the right by placing the corresponding letter in the space before the definition.

1. _____ Slight muscle paralysis

2. _____ Inflammation of a fascia

3. _____ Muscle disease

4. _____ Inflammation of a muscle

5. _____ Suture of a tendon

6. _____ Spasmodic involuntary twitching of a muscle that is normally under voluntary control

7. _____ Painful involuntary muscle spasm

8. _____ Rupture of a muscle

9. _____ Surgical repair of a tendon and muscle

10. _____ Strain of the flexor muscles of the toes with pain along the tibia

A. Cramp
B. Fascitis
C. Myoparesis
D. Myopathy
E. Myorrhexis
F. Myositis
G. Shin splint
H. Tenomyoplasty
I. Tenorrhaphy
J. Tic

Write the meaning of the following abbreviations.

11. _____ ACL

12. _____ LOS

13. _____ EMG

14. _____ MS

15. _____ DTR

16. Spelling is important in scientific and medical applications because only one or two incorrect letters may change the meaning. For each of the following pairs of words, circle the one that is spelled correctly.

A. myosin   mysin   F. aponeurosis   aponurosis

B. myorexis   myorrhexis   G. synergist   sinergyst

C. diaphram   diaphragm   H. myparesis   myoparesis

D. acetylcholine   acetilcoline   I. sarcomere   sarcomeer

E. gastronemius   gastrocnemius   J. subthreshold   subthreshhold

17. Use these word parts to write terms that fit the given definitions.

-desis   myo-   -plasty   -tomy
fasci-   -pathy   -rraphy

A. _____   Any abnormal condition of skeletal muscle

B. _____   Suturing of torn fascia

C. _____   Surgical incision into, or division of, a muscle

D. _____   Suture of a fascia to skeletal attachment

E. _____   Surgical repair of a muscle

18. Write the meaning of the underlined portion of the word on the line following the word.

A. my<u>asthenia</u> gravis   _____

B. arthro<u>desis</u>   _____

C. <u>flex</u>ion   _____

D. <u>masse</u>ter muscle   _____

E. dia<u>phragm</u>   _____

F. <u>plant</u>algia   _____

G. myo<u>rrhexis</u>   _____

H. <u>sarc</u>oblast   _____

I. <u>myo</u>atrophy   _____

J. <u>delt</u>oid   _____

19. From your knowledge of word parts, write the meaning of each of the following words.

A. hyperactive   _____

B. bilateral   _____

C. kinesiology   _____

D. isometric   _____

E. plantalgia   _____

F. isotonic   _____

G. synarthrosis   _____

H. fibromyalgia   _____

I. abduction   _____

J. arthrodesis   _____

20. Ima Student's primary care practitioner prescribed a central-acting muscle relaxant to decrease some muscle spasms.

A. How do these drugs work? _____

B. List at least four side effects that may occur with these muscle relaxants. _____

TESTING COMPREHENSION

Multiple choice: Select the best response.

1. A bundle of muscle fibers is called (a) a fasciculus, (b) a motor unit, (c) a sarcomere, (d) an aponeurosis.

2. The cell membrane of a muscle cell is the (a) endomysium, (b) sarcolemma, (c) sarcoplasmic reticulum, (d) aponeurosis.

3. Within a muscle fiber, calcium ions are stored with the (a) T tubules, (b) sarcoplasmic reticulum, (c) myosin, (d) I bands.

4. In a sarcomere, the region where there is only actin fibers is the (a) I band, (b) A band, (c) H zone, (d) Z line.

5. The connective tissue covering around a fasciculus is the (a) sarcolemma, (b) endomysium; (c) epimysium, (d) perimysium.

6. The fixed, or stable, end of a muscle is the (a) origin, (b) belly, (c) gaster, (d) insertion.

7. Receptor sites for acetylcholine are located on the (a) sarcolemma, (b) sarcoplasmic reticulum, (c) synaptic cleft, (d) synaptic vesicles.

8. Events in skeletal muscle fiber contraction after a threshold impulse include (1) formation of cross bridges, (2) acetylcholine binds with receptors, (3) ATP binds with myosin, (4) calcium released into sarcoplasm, (5) power stroke, (6) myosin binding sites exposed. The correct sequence for these events is (a) 1, 3, 5, 2, 4, 6; (b) 3, 1, 4, 2, 5, 6; (c) 2, 4, 6, 1, 5, 3; (d) 1, 6, 2, 4, 3, 5.

9. The contraction strength of a muscle increases when there is a stronger stimulus. This is called (a) tetany, (b) motor unit summation, (c) wave summation, (d) treppe.

10. Increased contraction strength in response to repeated stimuli of the same intensity is (a) tetany, (b) wave summation, (c) muscle tone, (d) treppe.

11. When you lift a book off a desk, the type of contraction is (a) isotonic, (b) treppe, (c) isometric, (d) tone.

12. The energy to restore adenosine diphosphate (ADP) to ATP during muscle contraction initially comes from (a) creatine phosphate, (b) glucose, (c) fatty acids, (d) lactic acid.

13. Limited amounts of oxygen for aerobic respiration to supply ATP for muscle contractions is stored in (a) myosin heads, (b) actin filaments, (c) myoglobin, (d) creatine phosphate.

14. Jari is training for an upcoming marathon. She has no illusions of winning the race, but she wants to endure until she finishes the 26 miles. Which of the following is *not* correct about her energy source for muscle contractions during this extended race? (a) glucose and fatty acids become the primary energy source; (b) oxygen is required for the aerobic breakdown of glucose; (c) training for this race increases the efficiency with which oxygen is delivered to the muscle cells; (d) most of the ATP that is needed comes from anaerobic respiration.

15. The sternocleidomastoid muscle is named for its (a) shape, (b) action, (c) origin and insertion, (d) location.

16. Two sphincter muscles of facial expression are the (a) orbicularis oris and orbicularis oculi, (b) orbicularis oris and buccinator, (c) buccinator and zygomaticus, (d) orbicularis oculi and zygomaticus.

17. There are four muscles of mastication. All of them insert on the (a) temporal bone, (b) mandible, (c) sphenoid bone, (d) maxillae.

18. The movement required to decrease the angle between the arm and forearm is (a) extension, (b) adduction, (c) pronation, (d) flexion.

19. Lonnie was showing his two young children how to swing sparklers in arcs to make light patterns. They held the sparklers in their hands, and their arms made large conelike motions. This type of movement is (a) abduction, (b) pronation, (c) circumduction, (d) eversion.

20. The deepest muscle in the abdominal wall is the (a) internal oblique, (b) transverses abdominis, (c) rectus abdominis, (d) linea alba.

21. When the anatomy teacher asked Bozo a question, he shrugged his shoulder and mumbled, "I don't know." The muscle used to elevate the scapula when he shrugged his shoulder was the (a) trapezius, (b) deltoid, (c) latissimus dorsi, (d) pectoralis major.

22. Terrence was pitching in the final game of the season for his college's baseball team when he sustained a shoulder injury. The team physician diagnosed it as a torn rotator cuff. This injury involved the (a) deltoid muscle, (b) trapezius muscle, (c) triceps brachii muscle, (d) supraspinatus muscle.

23. Shasta loves horses and rides nearly every morning before going to classes at the local college. The thigh muscles she uses to stay on the horse, the horse rider's muscles, are the (a) gluteus maximus, (b) vastus medialis, (c) adductor magnus, (d) tensor fasciae latae.

24. Sean played football for his college's varsity team. During one game he made a spectacular catch, ran a few yards, then stumbled and fell over the goal line for a touchdown. The fans went wild until they realized their player was still down. Finally he was helped off the field. The diagnosis: a pulled hamstring. The muscle most likely involved in this injury was the (a) rectus femoris, (b) biceps femoris, (c) sartorius, (d) vastus lateralis.

25. After classes at her local college, Kari studies ballet at a dance studio because it helps her relax and build good muscle tome and balance. At times it appears she is dancing on her toes. Of the following, the muscle that keeps her "on her toes" is the (a) peroneus, (b) tibialis anterior, (c) sartorius, (d) gastrocnemius.

A STEP BEYOND

Go a step beyond the ordinary and learn more about a topic that is related to this chapter but not discussed in detail in the textbook. Select one of the following topics, or one suggested by your instructor, and write a brief paper (250 words minimum), create a poster, or develop a short presentation (approximately 4 to 5 minutes) that focuses on your selection. Suggested topics for this chapter include the following:

1. *Exercise.* What effect does exercise have on skeletal muscles? Compare the features and benefits of strengthening-type exercise with endurance type exercise.
2. *Lyme disease.* What is Lyme disease? What are the causes, stages, signs and symptoms, diagnosis, and treatment?
3. *Joint replacement.* As they grow older, many people need to have knee replacements or hip replacements. Select either the knee or the hip and learn about the replacement procedure and the prosthetic device.

FUN & GAMES

World Scramble

Determine the word that fits each definition, then write the word in the spaces below the definition, one letter per space. The letters in the boxes form a scrambled word or words. Unscramble the letters to create a word or words that matches the final definition in each section.

1. Characteristic of muscles

2. Connective tissue around individual muscle fibers

3. Functional unit of a myofibril

4. Broad, flat sheet of tendon

Letters to use for final word: _____

Final definition: Surgical repair of a tendon and muscle

_____

5. Protein in thick filaments

6. Minimal stimulus to cause muscle fiber contraction

7. Principal muscle in the cheek

8. One of the muscles of mastication

Letters to use for final word: _____

Final definition: Transmitter at the neuromuscular junction

_____

8 Nervous System

LEARNING EXERCISES

Functions and Organization of the Nervous System

1. The two components of the CNS are the _____ and _____.

2. The two divisions of the peripheral nervous system are the _____, or sensory division, and the _____, or motor division.

3. The autonomic nervous system is a part of the _____ division of the peripheral nervous system.

4. The activities of the nervous system are grouped into three functional categories. These are _____, _____, and _____.

Nerve Tissue

1. Write the terms that fit the following descriptive phrases about neurons.

   A. _____   Process that conducts impulses toward the cell body

   B. _____   Fatty substance around some axons

   C. _____   Neurons that carry impulses toward the CNS

   D. _____   Gaps in the fatty substance around axons

   E. _____   Neurons entirely within the CNS

   F. _____   Conducts impulses away from the cell body

   G. _____   Has important role in nerve fiber regeneration

2. Write the name of the neuroglial cell that best fits each descriptive phrase.

   A. _____   Binds blood vessels to nerves

   B. _____   Phagocytic

   C. _____   Produces myelin within the CNS

   D. _____   Facilitates circulation of CSF

   E. _____   Supports cell bodies within ganglia

Nerve Impulses

1. Two functional characteristics of neurons are _____ and _____.

2. At rest, the outside of a neuron is _____ (charge) and has a higher concentration of _____ ions relative to the inside. A stimulus changes the permeability of the membrane and it depolarizes. During depolarization, _____ ions diffuse into the cell. This creates an _____ potential, or nerve impulse. During repolarization, _____ ions diffuse out of the cell. At the conclusion of the _____, the _____ pump restores the ionic conditions of a resting membrane. The minimum stimulus required to initiate a nerve impulse is called a _____ stimulus.

3. Match each of the following terms with the correct descriptive phrase.

convergence   inhibitory   refractory period
divergence   neurotransmitter   saltatory
excitatory   reflex arc   synapse

A. _____ Rapid conduction from node to node

B. _____ Region of communication between two neurons

C. _____ Diffuses across synaptic cleft

D. _____ Time during which a neuron is recovering from depolarization

E. _____ Synaptic transmission that initiates an impulse on the postsynaptic membrane

F. _____ Functional unit of the nervous system

G. _____ Single neuron synapses with multiple neurons

H. _____ Synaptic transmission that makes it more difficult to generate an impulse

I. _____ Several neurons synapse with a single postsynaptic neuron

4. Arrange the following numbered elements of a reflex arc in the correct sequence, beginning with the application of a stimulus, by writing the numbers in the appropriate order on the line provided: (1) axon of interneuron; (2) axon of motor neuron; (3) axon of sensory neuron; (4) cell body of interneuron; (5) cell body of motor neuron; (6) cell body of sensory neuron; (7) dendrite of interneuron; (8) dendrite of motor neuron; (9) dendrite of sensory neuron; (10) effector; (11) sensory receptor; (12) synapse between interneuron and motor neuron; (13) synapse between interneuron and sensory neuron.

_____ _____ _____ _____ _____ _____ _____ _____ _____ _____ _____ _____ _____

Central Nervous System

1. Arrange the following spaces and CNS coverings in the correct sequence by placing numbers 1–6 on the lines provided. Use 1 for the **outermost** and 6 for the **innermost.** Circle the space that is the location of CSF.

_____ Arachnoid   _____ Subarachnoid space   _____ Pia mater

_____ Epidural space   _____ Dura mater   _____ Subdural space

2. Write the name of the CNS structure that test fits each descriptive phrase.

A. _____ Second largest portion of the brain

B. _____ Includes the midbrain, pons, and medulla oblongata

C. _____ Includes the thalamus and hypothalamus

D. _____ Extends from the foramen magnum to the pons

E. _____ Diencephalon region regulating visceral activities

F. _____ Contains the apneustic and pneumotaxic centers

G. _____ Superior portion of the brainstem

H. _____ Coordinates skeletal muscles, posture, and balance

I. _____ Contains cardiac, vasomotor, respiratory centers

J. _____ Middle portion of the brainstem

3. Arrange the following numbered items in the appropriate sequence to represent the correct order of flow for CSF. Write the numbers in the appropriate order on the line provided:

(1) Openings in the fourth ventricle; (2) interventricular foramen; (3) Subarachnoid space; (4) fourth ventricle; (5) superior sagittal sinus; (6) Third ventricle; (7) choroid plexus of lateral ventricle; (8) arachnoid granulations; (9) cerebral aqueduct

_____ _____ _____ _____ _____ _____ _____ _____ _____

4. Each of the following statements about the spinal cord is false. Rewrite each statement to make it true.
   A. The spinal cord consists of a central core of white matter surrounded by gray matter.

   _____

   B. Two enlargements of the spinal cord are in the thoracic and lumbar regions.

   _____

   C. Ascending tracts carry motor impulses to the brain.

   _____

   D. Corticospinal tracts are ascending tracts that begin in the cerebral cortex.

   _____

Peripheral Nervous System

1. Within a nerve, each individual nerve fiber has a connective tissue covering called _____.

   The nerve itself is covered by connective tissue called _____.

2. Name the following cranial nerves.

   A. _____   Three nerves that are sensory only (3)

   _____

   _____

   B. _____   Nerve to the muscles of facial expression

   C. _____   Three nerves that function in eye movement

   _____

   _____

   D. _____   Nerve that is likely to be involved if you have a toothache in the lower jaw

   E. _____   Nerve to the muscles of mastication

   F. _____   Nerve that allows you to nod your head

3. Write the term or number that best fits each descriptive phrase.

   A. _____   Number of spinal nerves

   B. _____   Spinal nerve root that contains only sensory fibers

   C. _____   Complex network of nerve fibers

   D. _____   Number of cervical nerves

   E. _____   Spinal nerve root that contains only motor fibers

   F. _____   Nerve plexus that supplies nerves to the arm

   G. _____   Nerve plexus that gives rise to the phrenic nerve

   H. _____   Nerve plexus that gives rise to the sciatic nerve

4. The following table indicates some features of the autonomic nervous system. Use a check (√) to show which division of the autonomic nervous system is involved with each feature. Both divisions may be involved in some features and both columns should be checked.

S = Sympathetic division; P = Parasympathetic division.

Feature	S	P
A. Arises from thoracic and lumbar regions of the spinal cord		
B. Has terminal ganglia		
C. Also called the craniosacral division		
D. Has short preganglionic fibers		
E. Also called "fight-or flight"		
F. Cholinergic preganglionic fibers		
G. Adrenergic preganglionic fibers		
H. Also called "rest-and-repose" system		
I. Dilates pupils of the eyes		
J. Has short postganglionic fibers		
K. Increases heart rate		
L. Cholinergic postganglionic fibers		
M. Dilates blood vessels to skeletal muscles		
N. Increases digestive enzymes		
O. Constricts the bronchi		

LABELING AND COLORING EXERCISES

1. In Figure 8-1, color the cell body blue and the nucleus yellow. Label other components as indicated.

A. _____

B. _____

C. _____

D. _____

E. _____

F. _____

G. _____

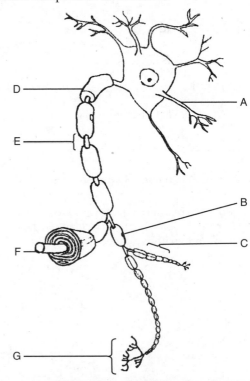

Figure 8-1 Typical neuron.

109

2. Figure 8-2 shows a midsagittal view of the brain. Label the regions as indicated. Color the somatosensory gyrus red, the somatomotor gyrus blue, the visual area green, and the brainstem yellow.

A. _____

B. _____

C. _____

D. _____

E. _____

F. _____

G. _____

H. _____

I. _____

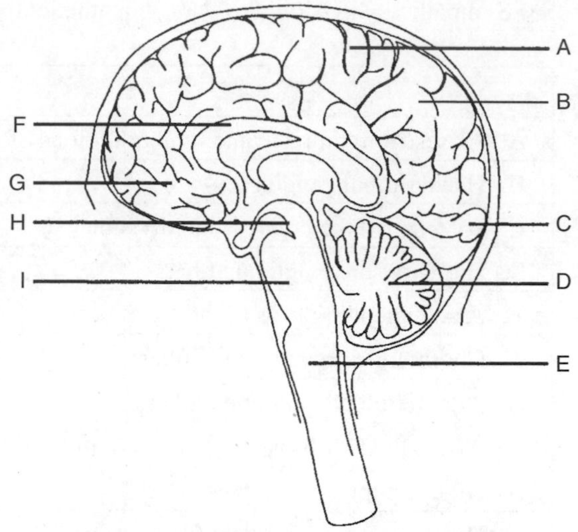

Figure 8-2   Midsagittal view of the brain.

3. Identify the parts of a spinal cord and spinal nerve that are indicated by leader lines in Figure 8-3 by writing the correct letter in the space provided before each term.

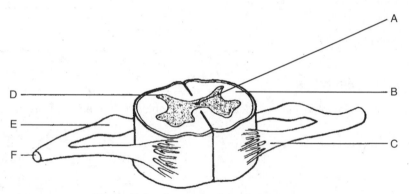

Figure 8-3   Cross section of spinal cord.

_____ Central canal   _____ Spinal nerve

_____ Dorsal horn   _____ Dorsal root ganglion

_____ Column of white matter   _____ Ventral root

4. Two types of efferent pathways are illustrated below. (a) Color the arrow(s) of the somatic motor pathway red and the autonomic pathway blue; (b) identify the arrows that represent preganglionic and postganglionic fibers by writing the words in the arrow space; (c) put an asterisk (*) by the effector that represents smooth muscle, cardiac muscle, and glands.

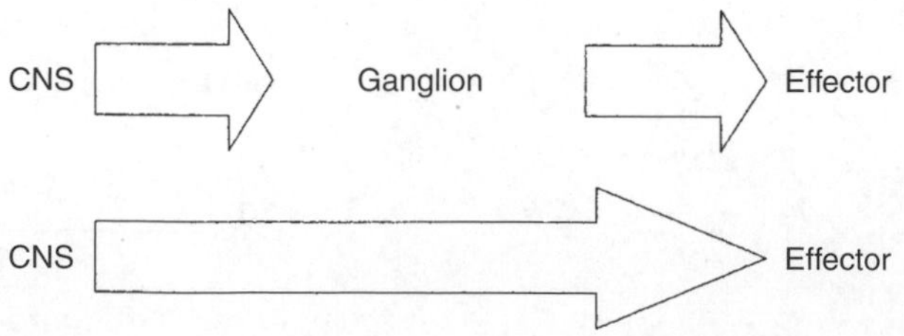

CNS   Ganglion   Effector

CNS   Effector

1. What are three types of functions performed by the nervous system?

    _____

2. What are the two main divisions of the nervous system, and how are these subdivided?

    _____

    _____

3. What two types of cells are found in nerve tissue?

    _____

4. What are the three basic parts of a neuron?

    _____

5. Draw a typical multipolar neuron and label the seven components.

6. What are the three functional types of neurons? How are they similar, and how are they different?

    _____

    _____

    _____

7. What is the function of neuroglia cells? How many types are there?

    _____

    _____

8. What are the two functional characteristics of neurons?

    _____

    _____

9. What is meant by the term *resting potential*? _____

    _____

10. What happens to the neuron cell membrane when a stimulus is applied? What is an action potential?

    _____

    _____

    _____

11. How are resting conditions restored after an action potential?

_____

12. What is meant by *threshold stimulus*?

_____

13. What is a *propagated action potential*?

_____

14. What is the advantage of saltatory conduction?

_____

_____

15. Diagram the components of a synapse, and describe how an impulse is conducted from one neuron to the next.

_____

_____

_____

16. What effect does an excitatory neurotransmitter have on the postsynaptic cell membrane? How does this differ from the effect of an inhibitory neurotransmitter?

_____

_____

_____

_____

17. How does a convergence circuit differ from a divergence circuit?

_____

_____

18. Diagram a reflex arc showing the five basic components.

19. What are the three different meninges, and what is their function?

_____

_____

_____

20. What are the five main regions or lobes of the cerebral hemispheres?

_____

_____

21. What are basal ganglia, and where are they located?

_____

_____

22. Where are each of the following located? (a) primary sensory area; (b) primary motor area; (c) visual cortex; (d) auditory area.

_____

_____

_____

23. Where is the diencephalon? What are its component parts and what are their functions?

_____

_____

_____

_____

24. What are the three parts of the brainstem, and what are their functions?

_____

_____

_____

_____

25. What three vital reflex centers are located in the medulla oblongata?

_____

26. What is the function of the cerebellum?

_____

_____

27. What is CSF (cerebrospinal fluid)? Where is it produced? How does it circulate?

_____

_____

_____

28. How does the arrangement of gray and white matter in the spinal cord differ from that in the cerebrum? What are the functions of the gray and white matter in the spinal cord?

_____

_____

_____

29. What are the three connective tissue wrappings associated with a nerve?

_____

_____

30. What are the names of the 12 cranial nerves, and what is the function of each one?

_____

_____

_____

_____

_____

_____

_____

_____

_____

_____

_____

31. What are the structure and function of spinal nerves? How many are there? How are they grouped?

_____

_____

_____

32. What is a nerve plexus?

_____

33. How do the pathways in the autonomic nervous system differ from somatic efferent pathways?

_____

34. What are the two major divisions of the autonomic nervous system? How do they differ in structure, function, and neurotransmitters?

_____

_____

_____

FUNCTIONAL RELATIONSHIPS

It is important to remember that no system in the body works alone. It takes the interaction of all systems to maintain homeostasis. The following exercises reinforce the concept that all systems work together to maintain the health and wellbeing of other systems and the individual.

Match the system on the right with what it provides for the nervous system on the left. Use the functional relationships page in your concepts textbook as a resource.

1. _____ Delivers oxygen and nutrients to the brain and spinal cord

2. _____ Provides protection for peripheral nerves and supports peripheral receptors

3. _____ Produces hormones that influence CNS development and sexual behavior

4. _____ Assists in defense against pathogens and in repair after trauma

5. _____ Protects brain and spinal cord

6. _____ Provides heat to maintain appropriate temperature for neural function

7. _____ Influences neural metabolism

8. _____ Absorbs nutrients for neural growth and metabolism

9. _____ Takes in oxygen for the neural tissue and helps maintain pH

10. _____ Eliminates metabolic wastes and helps maintain pH for neural function

A. Cardiovascular
B. Digestive
C. Endocrine
D. Integumentary
E. Lymphatic
F. Muscular
G. Reproductive
H. Respiratory
I. Skeletal
J. Urinary

For each of the following systems, write what the nervous system provides for it.

11. Cardiovascular _____

12. Skeletal _____

13. Reproductive _____

14. Endocrine _____

15. Respiratory _____

16. Muscular _____

17. Lymphatic _____

18. Digestive _____

19. Urinary _____

20. Integumentary _____

REPRESENTATIVE DISORDERS

Match the disorder of the skeletal system on the right with its description of the left.

A. _____ Congenital disorder with cranial vault and cerebral hemispheres missing

B. _____ Inflammation of the brain

C. _____ Blocks cholinesterase activity at the synapse

D. _____ Disrupted blood supply to the brain

E. _____ A type of senile dementia

F. _____ Bruising of brain tissue; signs persist more than 24 hours

G. _____ Abnormal accumulation of CSF within the ventricles

H. _____ Vertebral laminae do not close around spinal cord

I. _____ Caused by a bacterial toxin that attacks the CNS

J. _____ Inflammation of the meninges

1. Alzheimer disease
2. Anencephaly
3. Contusion
4. Encephalitis
5. Hydrocephalus
6. Meningitis
7. Nerve gas
8. Spina bifida
9. Stroke
10. Tetanus

VOCABULARY PRACTICE

1. Match the definitions on the left with the correct clinical term from the column on the right by placing the corresponding letter in the space before the definition.

A. _____ Used in the treatment of migraine headaches

B. _____ White, fatty substance around some nerve fibers

C. _____ Antiparkinsonism agent

D. _____ Lou Gehrig disease

E. _____ Nerve impulse

F. _____ Contains visual cortex

G. _____ Painful disorder of cranial nerve V

H. _____ Contains pneumotaxic and apneustic centers

I. _____ Contains the primary somatomotor cortex

J. _____ Contains cardiac, vasomotor, and respiratory centers

1. Action potential
2. ALS
3. Carbidopa-levodopa
4. Dihydroergotamine
5. Frontal lobe
6. Medulla oblongata
7. Myelin
8. Occipital lobe
9. Pons
10. Tic douloureux

2. Write the meaning of the following abbreviations.

A. _____ CVA   F. _____ TIA

B. _____ EEG   G. _____ ICP

C. _____ CSF   H. _____ PNS

D. _____ ADD   I. _____ LP

E. _____ CT   J. _____ PET

3. Spelling is important in scientific and medical applications because only one or two incorrect letters may change the meaning. For each of the following pairs of words, circle the one that is spelled correctly.

A. synapse   sinapse   F. dendrite   dendryte

B. ponds   pons   G. threshhold   threshold

C. neurolemma   neurilemma   H. thalmus   thalamus

D. sclerosis   sclairosis   I. mammilary   mamillary

E. trigiminal   trigeminal   J. pneumotaxic   newmotaxic

4. Write the meaning of the underlined portion of each word on the line preceding the word.

A. _____ schizophrenia

B. _____ epilepsy

C. _____ narcolepsy

D. _____ analgesic

E. _____ glossopharyngeal

F. _____ plexus

G. _____ meninges

H. _____ anesthesia

I. _____ insomnia

J. _____ dendrite

5. Use these word parts to write clinical terms that fit the given definitions.

encephal-   hyper-   myel-   -pathy
-gram   -itis   neur-   -plasty

A. _____   Inflammation of the brain

B. _____   Surgical repair of a nerve

C. _____   Inflammation of the spinal cord

D. _____   Any degenerative disease of the brain

E. _____   Record of a study of the spinal cord

6. For each of the following words, underline the word part that corresponds to the underlined word or phrase in the definition.

A. afferent   conducting toward a center

B. contralateral   pertaining to or affecting the opposite side

C. insomnia   inability to sleep

D. narcotic   a drug that induces stupor or sleep

E. anesthesia   without feeling

F. idiopathic   self originating; occurring without a known cause

G. kleptomania   obsessive preoccupation with stealing

H. aphasia   without speech

I. quadriplegia   paralysis of all four extremities

J. ganglion   a group or knot of nerve cell bodies

TESTING COMPREHENSION

Multiple choice: Select the best response.

1. Which of the following are components of the CNS? (a) brain and cranial nerves, (b) cranial nerves and spinal verves, (c) spinal cord and spinal nerves, (d) brain and spinal cord.

2. The afferent portion of a neuron is (a) a dendrite, (b) an axon, (c) a telodendria, (d) an axon collateral.

3. The white fatty tissue around an axon is (a) the endoneurium, (b) myelin, (c) the cell membrane, (d) the neuroglia.

4. Cells that form myelin in the CNS are (a) astrocytes, (b) microglia, (c) oligodendrocytes, (d) ependymal cells.

5. Which of the following is a correct pairing of a neuroglial cell type and its function? (a) microglia/phagocytosis; (b) ependymal cells/bind blood vessels to nerves; (c) astrocytes/circulate CSF; (d) satellite cells/form myelin sheaths.

6. The following are events in the initiation of a action potential: (1) membrane becomes permeable to potassium, (2) threshold stimulus is applied, (3) sodium/potassium pump restores resting conditions, (4) inside of membrane is positive to the outside, (5) membrane becomes permeable to sodium, (6) membrane is polarized with potassium outside. What is the correct sequence for these events? (a) 2, 1, 4, 6, 5, 3; (b) 2, 3, 1, 6, 4, 5; (c) 2, 5, 3, 1, 4, 6; (d) 2, 5, 4, 1, 6, 3.

7. Saltatory conduction occurs (a) in the gray matter of the spinal cord; (b) in the gray matter of the cerebrum; (c) in the myelinated nerve fibers; (d) in unmyelinated nerve fibers.

8. Which of the following is *not* true about synaptic transmission? (a) neurotransmitters react with receptor sites on the postsynaptic membrane, (b) impulses jump across the synapse by saltatory conduction, (c) inhibitory neurotransmitters hyperpolarize the cell membrane, (d) excitatory neurotransmitters depolarize the postsynaptic membrane.

9. Thinking about food, smelling food, and seeing food all start the flow of saliva. This is an example of a (a) simple series circuit, (b) divergence circuit, (c) convergence circuit, (d) inhibitory transmission.

10. When several muscles must contract simultaneously, it is important that the same information goes along different pathways at the same time. This is an example of (a) an inhibitory transmission circuit, (b) divergence circuit, (c) simple series circuit, (d) convergence circuit.

11. The arachnoid is (a) the middle layer of meninges, (b) the location of the superior sagittal sinus, (c) more delicate than the pia mater, (d) made of myelin.

12. The somatosensory area is located in the (a) frontal lobe, (b) parietal lobe, (c) occipital lobe, (d) temporal lobe.

13. The central sulcus separates the (a) parietal lobe from the occipital lobe, (b) parietal lobe from the temporal lobe, (c) occipital lobe from the temporal lobe, (d) frontal lobe from the parietal lobe.

14. Basal ganglia are regions of gray matter scattered throughout the (a) diencephalon, (b) cerebellum, (c) brainstem, (d) cerebrum.

15. The largest portion of the diencephalon is the (a) thalamus, (b) pons, (c) arbor vitae, (d) corpora quadrigemina.

16. The extension of dura mater that separates the cerebrum from the cerebellum is the (a) falx cerebri, (b) falx cerebelli, (c) tentorium cerebelli, (d) diaphragm sellae.

17. CSF arises as a filtrate from the (a) arachnoid granulations, (b) ependymal cells, (c) choroid plexus, (d) superior sagittal sinus.

18. The spinal cord is anchored to the coccyx by an extension of the pia mater called the (a) filum terminale, (b) cauda equina (c) conus medullaris, (d) pyramidal tract.

19. In the spinal cord the gray matter (a) is superficial to white matter; (b) is separated into dorsal, lateral, and ventral horns; (c) is divided by a dorsal median fissure; (d) contains longitudinal bundles of myelinated fibers.

20. The three cranial nerves that contain only sensory fibers are the (a) optic, abducens, and facial; (b) olfactory, trochlear, and trigeminal; (c) trochlear, trigeminal, and vagus; (d) optic, olfactory, and vestibulocochlear.

21. Three cranial nerves involved in eye movements are the (a) accessory, abducens, and vagus; (b) oculomotor, abducens, and trochlear; (c) trochlear, trigeminal, and facial; (d) oculomotor, facial, and trigeminal.

22. Which one of the following is *not* a correctly matched pair of terms? (a) cervical plexus/phrenic nerve; (b) lumbosacral plexus/median nerve; (c) brachial plexus/radial nerve; (d) lumbosacral plexus/sciatic nerve.

23. Which one of the following does *not* pertain to the sympathetic nervous system? (a) short preganglionic fibers, (b) widespread and long-lasting effect, (c) shows little divergence, (d) adrenergic fibers.

119

24. The parasympathetic nervous system (a) is the craniosacral division, (b) has prevertebral ganglia, (c) has both cholinergic and adrenergic fibers, (d) has a localized effect that is long-lasting.

25 Stimulation of the thoracolumbar division of the autonomic nervous system (a) constricts the bronchi, (b) increases secretions of digestive enzymes, (c) constricts the pupil of the eye, (d) increases heart rate.

A STEP BEYOND

Go a step beyond the ordinary and learn more about a topic that is related to this chapter but not discussed in detail in the textbook. Select one of the following topics, or one suggested by your instructor, and write a brief paper (250 words minimum), create a poster, or develop a short presentation (approximately 4 to 5 minutes) that focuses on your selection. Suggested topics for this chapter include the following:

1. *Caffeine*. Learn about the effects of caffeine on the nervous system. Report what you learn.
2. *Alcohol*. Learn about the effects of alcohol on the nervous system. Report what you learn.
3. *Ritalin*. What is Ritalin? What does it do? What effect does it have on the nervous system? For what conditions is it often prescribed? Investigate these questions and describe what you learn.
4. *Alzheimer disease*. A lot of attention is given to Alzheimer disease. What it is and how does it differ from other types of senile dementia? What happens in the nervous system that causes it? Learn about Alzheimer disease and describe what you learn.

FUN & GAMES

Word Scramble

Determine the word that fits each definition, and then write the word in the spaces below the definition, one letter per space. The letters in the boxes form a scrambled word or words. Unscramble the letters to create a word or words that matches the final definition in each section.

1. Part of the brain that includes the thalamus

2. Second largest part of the human brain

3. Region of communication between two neurons

4. Nerve impulse

Letters to use for final words: _____

Final definition: Process in which a nerve impulse travels along a myelinated fiber

_____

5. Nerve cells

6. Afferent processes of a nerve cell

7. Plays an important role in regeneration of nerve fibers

8. Body system that absorbs nutrients for synthesis for neurotransmitters

9. First cranial nerve

Letters to use for final words: _____

Final definition: Visceral efferent nerves

_____

9 Sensory System

LEARNING EXERCISES

Receptors and Sensations

1. Senses with receptors that are widely distributed within the body are called _____ senses. If the receptors are localized in a specific region, they are called _____ senses.

2. In the blank at the left, write the type of sense receptor that responds to the indicated stimulus.

   A. _____ Light energy

   B. _____ Changes in pressure or movement

   C. _____ Temperature changes

   D. _____ Tissue damage

   E. _____ Changes in chemical composition

3. _____ occurs when certain receptors are continually stimulated and no longer respond unless the stimulus becomes more intense.

General Senses

1. Place a check (✓) in the space before each correct association.

   A. _____ Pacinian corpuscles/mechanoreceptors

   B. _____ Pain/nociceptors

   C. _____ Mechanoreceptors/proprioception

   D. _____ Golgi tendon organs/touch

   E. _____ Meissner corpuscles/heavy pressure

2. Circle the word in the parentheses that makes the statement true.

   A. (Thermoreceptors/Nociceptors) exhibit rapid sensory adaptation.

   B. (Proprioceptors/Nociceptors) may send impulses after the stimulus is removed.

Gustatory Sense

1. Write the terms that best fit the following descriptive phrases.

    A. _____   Another name for sense of taste

    B. _____   Projections on tongue that contain taste buds

    C. _____   Structures that project through a taste pore

    D. _____   Type of receptors involved in taste

2. Write the terms that best fit the following descriptive phrases about taste.

    A. _____   Four types of taste sensations

    _____

    _____

    _____

    B. _____   Transmits impulses from anterior tongue

    C. _____   Transmits impulses from posterior tongue

    D. _____   Location of sensory cortex for taste in brain

Olfactory Sense

1. The chemoreceptors for olfaction are found in the olfactory epithelium located in the _____.

2. The olfactory nerve, cranial nerve number _____, transmits impulses to the olfactory cortex in the _____ lobe of the brain.

3. Airborne molecules may stimulate the sense of _____ and the sense of _____ at the same time.

Visual Sense

1. Write the terms that best fit the following descriptive phrases about the eye.

    A. _____   Gland that produces tears

    B. _____   Mucous membrane that lines the eyelid

    C. _____   White part of the fibrous tunic

    D. _____   Anterior transparent part of the fibrous tunic

    E. _____   Pigmented vascular tunic

    F. _____   Opening in the center of the iris

    G. _____   Fluid in the anterior cavity of the eye

H. _____ Muscles that regulate size of the pupil

I. _____ Muscles that control shape of the lens

J. _____ Function of the ciliary processes

K. _____ Nervous tunic of the eye

L. _____ Photoreceptor cells

M. _____ Region where the optic nerve penetrates the eye

N. _____ Depression in the center of the macula lutea

O. _____ Gel-like fluid in the posterior cavity

2. In the normal eye, light rays from distant objects are bent so they focus on the retina. This bending of light rays is called _____ .

3. Circle the correct word in each pair to make true statements. Accommodation is the adjustment needed to focus light rays for (distant/close) vision. To focus light rays from close objects, the ciliary muscle (relaxes/contracts), which (increases/decreases) the tension on the suspensory ligaments. When this happens, the lens becomes (thicker/thinner) and light rays are bent (more/less). In addition, the pupil (dilates/constricts).

4. Write the terms that best fit the following descriptive phrases about photoreceptors.

A. _____ Receptors for bright light vision

B. _____ Pigment contained in rods

C. _____ Receptors for color vision

D. _____ Colors of light absorbed by color receptors

E. _____ Receptors for dim light vision

F. _____ Pigment that is very light-sensitive

G. _____ Receptors not present in the fovea

H. _____ Vitamin required for photopigment synthesis

I. _____ Area of retina lacking photoreceptors

J. _____ Photoreceptors that exhibit greater convergence

5. Use the numbers 1 through 7 in the blanks to indicate the order of impulse transmission in the visual pathway. Use number 1 for the origination of the impulse and number 7 for the final visual cortex.

_____ Optic chiasma   _____ Optic tract   _____ Photoreceptors   _____ Optic nerve

_____ Thalamus   _____ Optic radiations   _____ Occipital lobe

Auditory Sense

1. Write the terms that best fit the following descriptive phrases about the inner ear.

A. _____ Series of interconnecting chambers in temporal bone

B. _____ Membranous tubes inside bony labyrinth

C. _____ Fluid inside the membranous labyrinth

D. _____ Fluid outside the membranous labyrinth

E. _____ Coiled portion of bony labyrinth

F. _____ Coiled portion of membranous labyrinth

G. _____ Membrane upon which the organ of Corti rests

H. _____ Membrane between scala vestibuli and cochlear duct

I. _____ Membrane between scala tympani and cochlear duct

2. Complete the following sentences about the events in the initiation of auditory impulses by writing the correct words in the spaces on the left.

Sound waves travel through the external auditory meatus until they reach the $\underline{A}$, which starts to vibrate. These vibrations are transferred to the $\underline{B}$, then the $\underline{C}$, then the $\underline{D}$, which is attached to the oval window. The oval window passes the vibrations to the $\underline{E}$ in the scala vestibuli of the inner ear. As vibrations pass through the scala vestibuli, they create corresponding movement of the $\underline{F}$ within the scala media. Finally, the vibrations are transferred to the basilar membrane and as it moves up and down, the $\underline{G}$ of the organ of Corti rub against the $\underline{H}$ and bend. This mechanical deformation initiates the nerve impulses that result in hearing. Pitch is determined by the region of the $\underline{I}$ that vibrates in response to the sound. Loudness is determined by magnitude of $\underline{J}$ of the membrane.

A. _____   F. _____

B. _____   G. _____

C. _____   H. _____

D. _____   I. _____

E. _____   J. _____

Sense of Equilibrium

1. Write the terms that best fit the following descriptive phrases about the sense of equilibrium.

A. _____ Equilibrium of rotational or angular movement

B. _____ Position of head relative to gravity

C. _____ Receptor organ for static equilibrium

D. _____ Chambers containing static equilibrium organs (2)

_____

E. _____ Calcium carbonate crystals on surface of the macula

F. _____ Receptor organ for dynamic equilibrium

G. _____ Location of dynamic equilibrium receptor organ

LABELING AND COLORING EXERCISES

Identify the listed structures of the bulbus oculi by matching them with the correct letters from the diagram in Figure 9-1. Color the two surfaces or structures that bend light rays red and color the two liquid media yellow.

1. _____ Anterior cavity   7. _____ Lens

2. _____ Choroid   8. _____ Optic nerve

3. _____ Ciliary body   9. _____ Posterior cavity

4. _____ Cornea   10. _____ Retina

5. _____ Eyelid   11. _____ Sclera

6. _____ Iris   12. _____ Suspensory ligaments

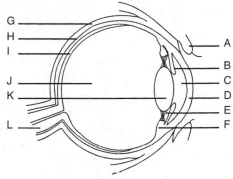

Figure 9-1 Bulbus oculi.

13. Figure 9-2 illustrates layers of the retina. Label structures and layers as indicated. Color the rods and cone layer blue, the bipolar neuron layer pink, and the ganglion layer yellow.

A. _____

B. _____

C. _____

D. _____

E. _____

F. _____

G. _____

H. _____

I. _____

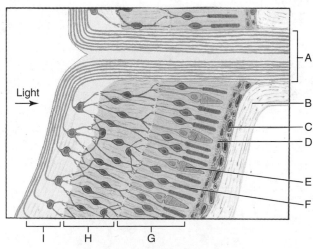

Figure 9-2 Retina of the eye.

Figure 9-3 illustrates the structure of the ear. Identify the structures indicated by matching them with the correct letter from the diagram. Color the region of the external ear red, middle ear yellow, and inner ear blue.

14. _____   Ampulla

15. _____   Auditory tube

16. _____   Auricle

17. _____   Cochlea

18. _____   External auditory canal

19. _____   Incus

20. _____   Malleus

21. _____   Semicircular canals

22. _____   Stapes

23. _____   Tympanic membrane

24. _____   Vestibule

25. _____   Vestibulocochlear nerve

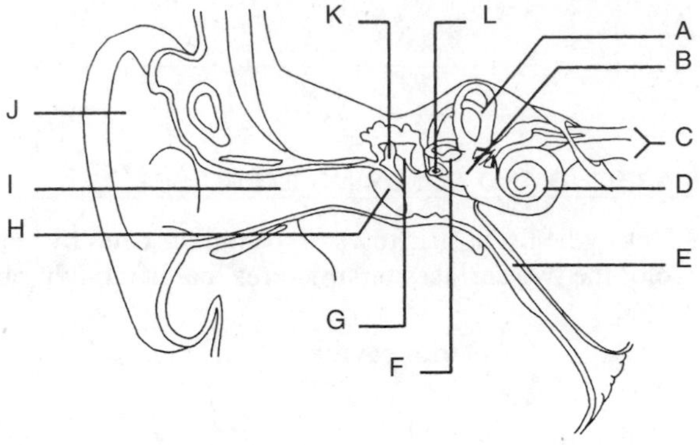

Figure 9-3   Structure of the ear.

26. Figure 9-4 illustrates a section through the cochlea. Identify the structures indicated. Color the region that contains endolymph yellow.

A. _____

B. _____

C. _____

D. _____

E. _____

F. _____

G. _____

H. _____

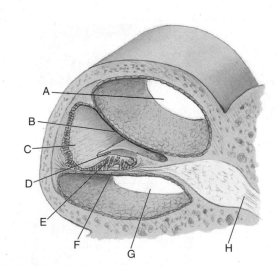

Figure 9-4   Section through the cochlea.

1. What is the difference in the distribution of the receptors for the general senses and the special senses?

   _____

   _____

2. What are the five classes of sense receptors?

   _____

   _____

   _____

   _____

   _____

3. What is meant by sensory adaptation?

   _____

   _____

4. Name three receptors involved in the sense of touch and pressure.

   _____

   _____

   _____

5. What term is given to the sense of position or orientation? Name two receptors involved with this sense.

   _____

   _____

6. What stimulates nociceptors?

   _____

7. Where are the receptors for taste located?

   _____

8. Name the four different types of taste.

   _____

   _____

   _____

   _____

9. What cranial nerve is involved in the sense of smell?

   _____

10. In what ways are the senses of taste and smell related?

_____

_____

11. What bones are in the orbit of the eye?

_____

_____

12. What is the function of eyelashes, eyelids, and eyebrows?

_____

_____

_____

13. Where are tears produced, and what is their function?

_____

_____

_____

_____

14. Draw and label a diagram that illustrates the three layers of the bulbus oculi.

15. Where are the aqueous humor and vitreous humor located?

_____

_____

16. What parts of the bulbus oculi bend light rays so they focus on the retina?

_____

_____

17. How does the ciliary body act to change the shape of the lens for accommodation?

_____

_____

18. What are the rods and cones, and where are they located?

_____

_____

19. How do photoreceptor cells trigger nerve impulses?

_____

_____

_____

_____

20. Which cranial nerve transmits visual impulses, and where are these impulses interpreted?

_____

_____

21. Draw and label a diagram of the ear.

22. What three bones are found in the ear?

_____

23. What fluid is found inside the bony labyrinth but outside the membranous labyrinth?

_____

24. In what specific portion of the ear are the auditory receptors located?

_____

25. How are sound vibrations converted into auditory impulses?

_____

_____

_____

_____

_____

26. How does the ear distinguish between loud sounds and soft or quiet sounds?

_____

_____

27. In what part of the brain is the auditory cortex located?

_____

28. What is the difference between *static equilibrium* and *dynamic equilibrium*?

_____

_____

_____

_____

29. Where are the receptors for static equilibrium located?

_____

_____

30. Where are the receptors for dynamic equilibrium located?

_____

_____

31. What mechanical event triggers impulses for equilibrium?

_____

32. Which cranial nerve transmits impulses for equilibrium to the central nervous system?

_____

REPRESENTATIVE DISORDERS

Match the disorder of the skeletal system on the right with its description of the left.

1. _____ Deviation of one eye form the other; cross-eyed

2. _____ Light rays focus in front of the retina

3. _____ Lack of sense of smell

4. _____ One sign is increased intraocular pressure

5. _____ Abnormal or perverted sense of taste

6. _____ Defective curvature of cornea or lens of the eye

7. _____ Swimmer's ear

8. _____ Otitis interna with dizziness and loss of balance

9. _____ Lens of the eye becomes opaque

10. _____ Involuntary, rapid movements of the eyeball

A. Anosmia

B. Astigmatism

C. Cataract

D. Glaucoma

E. Labyrinthitis

F. Myopia

G. Nystagmus

H. Otomycosis

I. Parageusia

J. Strabismus

VOCABULARY PRACTICE

Match the definitions on the left with the correct clinical term from the column on the right by placing the corresponding letter in the space before the definition. Not all terms will be used.

1. _____ Cause pupil dilation

2. _____ Responds to tissue damage

3. _____ Inflammation of the inner ear

4. _____ Impairment of hearing due to aging

5. _____ Paralyze ciliary muscle to prevent accommodation

6. _____ Fungal infection of the external ear

7. _____ Night blindness

8. _____ Ringing or buzzing sound in the ears

9. _____ Defective curvature of the cornea

10. _____ Characterized by increased intraocular pressure

A. Astigmatism

B. Cycloplegic agents

C. Emmetropia

D. Glaucoma

E. Labyrinthitis

F. Meniere disease

G. Mydriatic agents

H. Nociceptors

I. Nyctalopia

J. Otalgia

K. Otomycosis

L. Otosclerosis

M. Presbycusis

N. Tinnitus

11. Write the meaning of the following abbreviations.

A. _____ REM

B. _____ EOM

C. _____ EENT

D. _____ AOM

E. _____ IOL

F. _____ db

G. _____ POAG

H. _____ LASIK

I. _____ IOP

J. _____ AMD

12. Spelling is important in scientific and medical applications because only one or two incorrect letters can change the meaning. All of the following words are from this chapter, and six are spelled incorrectly. Place a (✓) in the space preceding the words that are spelled correctly, and write the correct spelling in the space preceding the misspelled words.

A. _____ eustachian   D. _____ lacrimal

B. _____ oldfactory   E. _____ retna

C. _____ gustatary   F. _____ prespyopia

G. _____ blefaritis   I. _____ diplopia

H. _____ otalgia   J. _____ midrysis

13. Write the meaning of the underlined portion of each word on the line preceding the word.

A. _____   blepharitis

B. _____   hyperopia

C. _____   phacoemulsification

D. _____   myringitis

E. _____   dacryolith

F. _____   dacryoadenalgia

G. _____   keratometer

H. _____   presbycusis

I. _____   vitreous

J. _____   lacrimation

14. Use these word parts to write clinical terms that fit the given definitions.

dacry-   irid-   myring-   oto-   -plasty
-ectomy   kerat-   -oma   -otomy

A. _____   Excision of a full-thickness piece of the iris

B. _____   Incision of the cornea

C. _____   Plastic surgery of the external ear

D. _____   Excision of the tympanic membrane

E. _____   Tumor-like swelling due to obstruction of the lacrimal duct

F. _____   Surgical repair of the tympanic membrane

G. _____   Incision into the iris

H. _____   Plastic surgery of the cornea

15. For each of the following words, underline the word part that corresponds to the underlined word or phrase in the definition.

A. cochlea   snail-shaped portion of the inner ear

B. dacryoadenalgia   pain in a lacrimal gland

C. macula lutea   yellow depression of the retina

D. presbyopia   impaired accommodation in <u>old age</u>

E. phacocele   hernia of the <u>eye lens</u>

F. ophthalmomycosis   a <u>fungal</u> disease of the eye

G. gustation   act of <u>tasting</u>

H. blepharectomy   surgical excision of an <u>eyelid</u>

I. fovea centralis   a small <u>pit</u> in the retina

J. olfactometer   an instrument for testing the sense of <u>smell</u>

TESTING COMPREHENSION

Multiple choice: Select the best response.

1. The sense of touch is (a) a general sense that utilizes thermoreceptors, (b) a general sense that utilizes mechanoreceptors, (c) a special sense that utilizes nociceptors, (d) a special sense that utilizes chemoreceptors.

2. Pain from a burn is (a) a special sense from thermoreceptors, (b) a special sense from mechanoreceptors, (c) a general sense from thermoreceptors, (d) a general sense from nociceptors.

3. Hearing is a (a) general sense from mechanoreceptors, (b) general sense from chemoreceptors, (c) special sense from chemoreceptors, (d) special sense from mechanoreceptors.

4. Which of the following is *not* correct about the sense of taste? (a) it is also called the gustatory sense; (b) in order to be tasted, substances must be dissolved; (c) receptors for the different tastes are randomly distributed over the surface of the tongue; (d) the facial and glossopharyngeal nerves transmit impulses for taste to the parietal lobe of the brain.

5. Which of the following is *not* correct about protective features of the eye? (a) the frontal, ethmoid, and zygomatic bones contribute to the bony socket of the eye; (b) the gland that produces tears is located along the upper medial margin of the eye; (c) tears contain an enzyme that helps destroy pathogenic bacteria; (d) sebaceous glands are associated with eyelashes.

6. The white portion of the outer tunic of the bulbus oculi is the (a) sclera, (b) cornea, (c) choroid, (d) conjunctiva.

7. The depression in the center of the macula lutea is the (a) optic disk and primarily contains rods, (b) optic disk and primarily contains cones, (c) fovea centralis and primarily contains rods, (d) fovea centralis and primarily contains cones.

8. The portion of the eye that contains muscles that change the size of the pupil is the (a) cornea, (b) ciliary body, (c) iris, (d) suspensory ligaments.

9. The region where the optic nerve exits the eye is the (a) optic disk, (b) macula lutea, (c) fovea centralis, (d) palpebrae.

10. The first portion of the eye that refracts light is the (a) lens, (b) cornea, (c) pupil, (d) aqueous humor.

11. The structure of the eye that has the greatest effect on accommodation is the (a) cornea, (b) pupil, (c) vitreous humor, (d) lens.

12. When the eyes accommodate for close vision, (a) the ciliary muscles relax, the suspensory ligaments are taut, and the lens is flat; (b) the ciliary muscles contract, the suspensory ligaments are taut, and the lens becomes convex; (c) the ciliary muscles contract, the suspensory ligaments are loose, and the lens is flat; (d) the ciliary muscles contract, the suspensory ligaments are loose, and the lens becomes convex.

133

13. Which of the following represents the correct sequence for the visual pathway? (a) optic tract, optic chiasma, optic nerve, thalamus, optic radiations, visual cortex; (b) optic radiations, optic tract, optic chiasma, optic nerve, thalamus, visual cortex; (c) optic nerve, optic chiasma, optic tract, thalamus, optic radiations, visual cortex; (d) optic nerve, thalamus, optic tract, optic chiasma, optic radiations, visual cortex.

14. The visual lobe is located in the (a) frontal lobe of the brain, (b) occipital lobe of the brain, (c) parietal lobe of the brain, (d) temporal lobe of the brain.

15. Lauren was having some difficulty with her vision, so she made an appointment with an ophthalmologist. The ophthalmologist diagnosed myopia and explained that in this condition (a) excess tears absorb light rays before they enter the cornea; (b) intraocular pressure increases and interferes with the refraction of light; (c) the light rays bend too much and focus in front of the retina; (d) the cornea has an irregular curvature and scatters the light rays.

16. Most of the ear is not visible because it is located within the (a) frontal bone, (b) temporal bone, (c) parietal bone, (d) maxilla.

17. Which one of the following parts of the ear is involved in the sense of equilibrium, but not involved in the sense of hearing? (a) semicircular canals, (b) cochlea, (c) endolymph, (d) organ of Corti.

18. Which one of the following parts of the ear is involved in the sense of hearing but is not involved in the sense of equilibrium? (a) semicircular canals; (b) hair cells; (c) tectorial membrane; (d) utricle and saccule.

19. The organ of Corti is located in the (a) scala vestibule, (b) scala tympani, (c) macula, (d) cochlear duct.

20. The malleus, incus, and stapes are located in the (a) external ear, (b) middle ear, (c) inner ear, (d) auricle.

21. Which one of the following is **not** associated with the middle ear? (a) eustachian tube, (b) ceruminous glands, (c) oval window, (d) auditory ossicles.

22. Which one of the following is associated with static equilibrium? (a) otoliths, (b) crista ampullaris, (c) semicircular canals, (d) incus.

23. The auditory cortex of the brain is located in the (a) thalamus, (b) medulla oblongata, (c) midbrain, (d) temporal lobe.

24. Which portion of the brain is especially important in mediating the sense of balance and equilibrium? (a) frontal lobe, (b) midbrain, (c) cerebellum, (d) diencephalon.

25. Luanne is concerned because her 3-year old son, Aaron, has frequent middle ear infections. The pediatrician explained that children are more susceptible to these infections than adults because children (a) get more water in their ears when taking a bath; (b) have a shorter and wider eustachian tube so bacteria get from the throat to the middle ear more readily; (c) put their dirty fingers into their ears and introduce bacteria; (d) have inactive ceruminous glands, so they have no cerumen to destroy bacteria.

A STEP BEYOND

Go a step beyond the ordinary and learn more about a topic that is related to this chapter but not discussed in detail in the textbook. Select one of the following topics, or one suggested by your instructor, and write a brief paper (250 words minimum), create a poster, or develop a short presentation (approximately 4 to 5 minutes) that focuses on your selection. Suggested topics for this chapter include the following:

1. *Macular degeneration*. Many people, as they age, develop macular degeneration. Compare the two types of this visual disorder, including their pathogenesis and prognosis.
2. *Glaucoma*. What is glaucoma? How does it develop? Is there a treatment? What is the prognosis? Report on what you learn.

3. *Deafness.* Compare conduction deafness with sensorineural deafness. What are the causes, pathogenesis, prognosis, and treatment?

4. *Motion sickness.* What is motion sickness? What causes it? Why are some people affected and others not? See what you can learn about motion sickness and report your findings.

FUN & GAMES

Word Scramble

Determine the word that fits each definition, and then write the word in the spaces across from the definition, one letter per space. The letters in the boxes form a scrambled word or words. Unscramble the letters to create a word or words that matches the final definition in each section.

1. Receptors for color vision

2. Impairment of vision caused by aging

3. Gel-like fluid in the posterior cavity of the eye

4. Malleus, incus, and stapes

Letters to use for final word: _____

Final definition: Fluid inside the membranous labyrinth

_____

5. Pain receptor

6. Hearing test

7. Portion of the vascular tunic of the eye

8. Region of the ear that includes the auricle

Letters to use for final word: _____

Final definition: Type of receptor for hearing

_____

10 Endocrine System

Introduction to the Endocrine System

For each of the following phrases, place an N in the space provided if the phrase pertains to the nervous system and an E if it pertains to the endocrine system.

1. _____ Acts through hormones

2. _____ Effect is localized

3. _____ Acts through electrical impulses

4. _____ Effect is of short-term duration

5. _____ Effect is generalized and long-term

6. Exocrine glands have _____ that carry the secretory product to a surface.

In contrast, _____ are ductless and secrete their product directly into the

_____ for transport to the target tissue.

Characteristics of Hormones

1. Write the terms that best fit the following descriptive phrases about the characteristics of hormones.

A. _____ Chemical nature of nonsteroid hormones

B. _____ Hormones that are lipid derivatives

C. _____ Cells that have hormone receptors

D. _____ Location of receptors for protein hormones

E. _____ Location of receptors for steroid hormones

F. _____ Mechanisms for controlling secretion (3)

_____

_____

2. Complete the following sentences about the reaction of a hormone with its receptor:

A <u>A</u> hormone combines with a receptor on the surface of the cell. This activates an enzyme within the membrane, called <u>B</u>, and the enzyme diffuses into the cytoplasm, where it catalyzes the production of <u>C</u>. This substance, a derivative of <u>D</u>, activates other enzymes that alter cellular activity. The <u>E</u> is called the first messenger, and <u>F</u> is called the second messenger. A <u>G</u> hormone diffuses through the cell membrane and reacts with a <u>H</u> within the cytoplasm. The complex that forms enters the <u>I</u> and reacts with <u>J</u> to stimulate protein synthesis.

A. _____   F. _____

B. _____   G. _____

C. _____   H. _____

D. _____   I. _____

E. _____   J. _____

Endocrine Glands and Their Hormones

1. Match each of the following phrases with the region of the pituitary gland that it describes.

A = adenohypophysis
N = neurohypophysis

A. _____   Secretes antidiuretic hormone (ADH)

B. _____   Stimulated by releasing hormones

C. _____   Secretes prolactin

D. _____   Derived from nervous tissue

E. _____   Secretes oxytocin

F. _____   Derived from embryonic oral cavity

G. _____   Secretes thyroid-stimulating hormone (FSH)

H. _____   Secretes growth hormone

I. _____   Secretes adrenocorticotropic hormone (ACTH)

J. _____   Regulated by nerve stimulation

2. Write the name of the pituitary hormones that best match the following functions.

A. _____   Stimulates secretion of thyroid hormone

B. _____   Stimulates the adrenal cortex

C. _____   Stimulates ovulation

D. _____   Stimulates uterine contractions

E. _____   Increases water reabsorption

F. _____ Stimulates spermatogenesis

G. _____ Stimulates protein synthesis and growth

H. _____ Stimulates ejection of milk

I. _____ Stimulates production of testosterone

J. _____ Stimulates milk production

3. Match each of the following phrases with the correct hormone from the thyroid and parathyroid glands.

C = calcitonin
P = parathyroid hormone
T = thyroxine

A. _____ Secreted by parafollicular cells

B. _____ Requires iodine for production

C. _____ Increases blood calcium levels

D. _____ Secreted by thyroid follicles

E. _____ Increases rate of metabolism

F. _____ Reduces blood calcium levels

G. _____ Increases osteoclast activity

H. _____ Hyposecretion leads to nerve excitability

4. Write the terms that best fit the following descriptive phrases about the adrenal gland.

A. _____ Region regulated by nerve impulses

B. _____ Group of hormones from the outer cortical layer

C. _____ Primary mineralocorticoid hormone

D. _____ Region regulated by negative feedback

E. _____ Primary glucocorticoid

F. _____ Increases blood sodium levels

G. _____ Counteracts inflammatory response

H. _____ Secreted by the innermost layer of the cortex

I. _____ Hormones from the adrenal medulla (2)

_____

5. Indicate whether each descriptive phrase refers to insulin (I) or to glucagon (G) by writing the appropriate letter in the space provided.

A. _____ Secreted in response to elevated blood glucose levels

B. _____ Secreted by the alpha cells

C. _____ Promotes breakdown of glycogen into glucose

D. _____ Secreted by the beta cells

E. _____ Stimulates liver to store glucose as glycogen

F. _____ Secreted in response to low blood glucose levels

G. _____ Increases blood glucose levels

H. _____ Decreases blood glucose levels

I. _____ Hyposecretion may result in diabetes mellitus

6. Each of the following hormones is preceded by two blanks. In the first blank, indicate the source of the hormone, and in the second blank, indicate a function of the hormone from the lists provided.

A. ____ ____ Testosterone	1. heart	A. alkaline fluid from pancreas
B. ____ ____ Melatonin	2. ovaries	B. contraction of gallbladder
	3. pineal gland	
C. ____ ____ Thymosin	4. placenta	C. decreases blood volume
D. ____ ____ Estrogen	5. small intestine	D. development of lymphocytes
E. ____ ____ HCG	6. stomach	E. female sex characteristics
	7. testes	
F. ____ ____ Gastrin	8. thymus	F. maintains pregnancy
G. ____ ____ Secretin		G. male sex characteristics
H. ____ ____ Progesterone		H. prepares uterus for pregnancy
I. ____ ____ Cholecystokinin		I. production of HCl in stomach
J. ____ ____ Atrial peptin		J. regulation of body rhythms

Prostaglandins

1. Prostaglandins are similar to hormones, but they are different in many ways. They are derivatives of

_____, and the cells that produce them are _____ through-

out the body.

2. In contrast to hormones, the effects of prostaglandins are _____,

_____, and _____.

1. Identify the endocrine glands shown in Figure 10-1 by writing the name of the gland in the corresponding space on the left.

A. _____

B. _____

C. _____

D. _____

E. _____

F. _____

G. _____

H. _____

I. _____

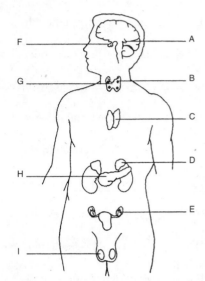

Figure 10-1 Major endocrine glands.

2. In Figure 10-2, color the adenohypophysis pink and the neurohypophysis yellow. Identify the hormones represented by the letters by writing the name and the abbreviation in the spaces provided.

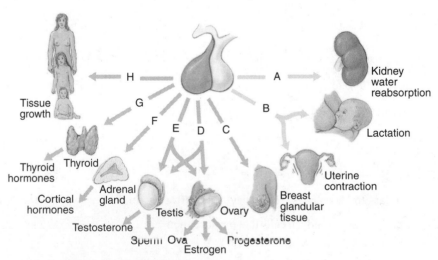

Figure 10-2 Effects of hormones from the pituitary gland.

A. _____

B. _____

C. _____

D. _____

E. _____

F. _____

G. _____

H. _____

3. Figure 10-3 illustrates the adrenal gland. Color the medulla pink and the cortex yellow. Identify the three classes of hormones that are secreted by the adrenal cortex and the two hormones that are secreted by the medulla.

Classes of hormones from the cortex:

A. _____

B. _____

C. _____

Hormones from the medulla:

D. _____

E. _____

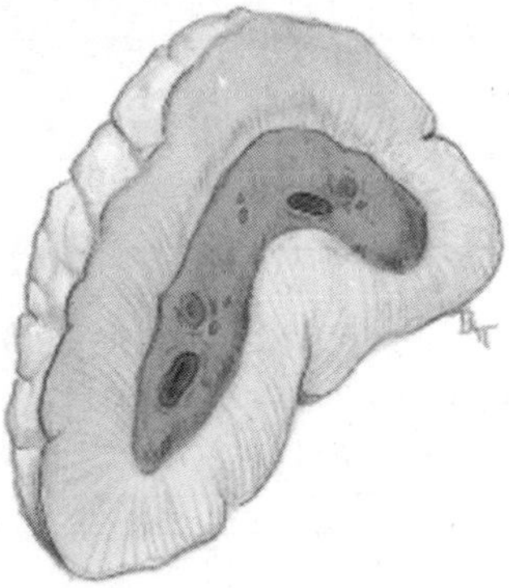

Figure 10-3   Adrenal gland.

REVIEW QUESTIONS

1. How does the endocrine system compare with the nervous system in its regulatory function?

_____

_____

_____

2. How do endocrine glands differ from exocrine glands in their mode of secretion?

_____

_____

_____

3. What are the two principal chemical classes of hormones?

_____

_____

4. How do hormones recognize their target tissues?

_____

_____

5. Where are the receptor sites for protein hormones located? Where are the receptor sites for steroid hormones located?

_____

_____

6. List three different mechanisms for regulating hormone secretion.

_____

7. How does a negative feedback system function to regulate hormone secretion?

_____

_____

_____

8. List the eight major endocrine glands.

_____

_____

9. How is the secretory activity of the adenohypophysis controlled? Neurohypophysis?

_____

_____

10. List six hormones secreted by the adenohypophysis.

_____

_____

11. For each of the six hormones secreted by the adenohypophysis, write a sentence that describes its action.

_____

_____

_____

_____

_____

12. What gland secretes ADH and oxytocin? What is the function of these two hormones?

_____

_____

_____

13. What portion of the thyroid gland secretes the hormones that contain iodine?

_____

14. What causes a simple goiter?

_____

_____

_____

15. What are the effects of hypersecretion and hyposecretion of thyroxine?

_____

_____

16. What is the function of calcitonin, and where is it produced?

_____

_____

_____

17. Where are the parathyroid glands located, and what is the function of the hormone they produce?

_____

_____

_____

18. How do calcitonin and parathyroid hormone differ in function?

_____

_____

_____

19. How do the adrenal cortex and medulla differ in the way their secretory activity is regulated?

_____

_____

_____

20. What hormones are produced by the adrenal cortex? What are their functions?

_____

_____

_____

_____

21. Which adrenocortical hormones are vital to life and why?

_____

_____

_____

22. What hormones have an effect that is similar to that of the sympathetic nervous system?

_____

23. What constitutes the endocrine portion of the pancreas?

_____

24. What cells produce glucagon? Insulin?

_____

_____

25. What is the difference in action between glucagon and insulin?

_____

_____

26. What is the main source of testosterone?

_____

27. What two hormones are produced by the ovaries?

_____

28. What two functions are attributed to melatonin?

_____

_____

_____

29. Of what importance is the thymus gland?

_____

_____

30. How do prostaglandins differ from hormones?

_____

_____

_____

31. What are some of the functions of prostaglandins?

_____

_____

_____

FUNCTIONAL RELATIONSHIPS

It is important to remember that no system in the body works alone. It takes the interaction of all systems to maintain homeostasis. The following exercises reinforce the concept that all systems work together to maintain the health and well-being of other systems and the individual. Match the system on the right with what it provides for the endocrine system on the left. Use the functional relationships page in your concepts textbook as a resource.

1. _____ Barrier against pathogen entry

2. _____ Helps maintain pH for endocrine metabolism

3. _____ Protects glands in head

4. _____ Produces hormones that regulate gonadotropins

5. _____ Provides protection for thyroid gland

6. _____ Eliminates inactivated hormones

7. _____ Transports hormones to target tissue

8. _____ Regulates activity of adrenal medulla

9. _____ Absorbs nutrients for hormone synthesis

10. _____ Defense against infection in endocrine glands

A. Cardiovascular
B. Digestive
C. Integumentary
D. Lymphatic
E. Muscular
F. Nervous
G. Reproductive
H. Respiratory
I. Skeletal
J. Urinary

For each of the following systems, write what the endocrine system provides for it.

11. Cardiovascular _____

12. Skeletal _____

13. Reproductive _____

14. Nervous _____

15. Respiratory _____

16. Muscular _____

17. Lymphatic _____

18. Digestive _____

19. Urinary _____

20. Integumentary _____

REPRESENTATIVE DISORDERS

Match the disorder of the endocrine system on the right with its description of the left.

1. _____ Excessive size and stature

2. _____ Deficiency of ADH with polyuria

3. _____ Enlargement of extremities

4. _____ Dwarfism with mental retardation

5. _____ Insufficient hormones from adrenal cortex

6. _____ Caused by high levels of cortisol

7. _____ Insufficient growth hormone in children

8. _____ Deficiency of pancreatic beta cell hormone

A. Acromegaly
B. Addison disease
C. Cretinism
D. Cushing syndrome
E. Diabetes insipidus
F. Diabetes mellitus
G. Dwarfism
H. Gigantism

VOCABULARY PRACTICE

Match the definitions on the left with the correct clinical term from the column on the right by placing the corresponding letter in the space before the definition. Not all terms will be used.

1. _____ Synthetic glucocorticoid

2. _____ Derived from arachidonic acid

3. _____ Premature aging that occurs in childhood

4. _____ Caused by a deficient quantity of ADH

5. _____ Used to treat decreased activity of the thyroid

6. _____ Excessive thirst

7. _____ Caused by excessive growth hormone in adult

8. _____ Posterior portion of the pituitary gland

9. _____ Tumor of a gland

10. _____ A group of symptoms caused by prolonged exposure to high levels of cortisol

A. Acromegaly
B. Adenohypophysis
C. Adenoma
D. Cushing syndrome
E. Diabetes insipidus
F. Diabetes mellitus
G. Levothyroxine sodium
H. Myxedema
I. Neurohypophysis
J. Polydipsia
K. Polyphagia
L. Prednisone
M. Prostaglandins
N. Progeria

11. Write the meaning of the following abbreviations.

A. ACTH _____

B. ADH _____

C. FBS _____

D. FSH _____

E. IDDM _____

F. PBI _____

G. TFT _____

H. GTT _____

I. T_3 _____

J. OXT _____

12. Spelling is important in scientific and medical applications because only one or two incorrect letters can change the meaning. All of the following words are from this chapter and are spelled incorrectly. Write the correct spelling in the space preceding the misspelled words.

A. _____ epinefrin   F. _____ hypofisis

B. _____ hydrocloric   G. _____ oxitosin

C. _____ natrietic   H. _____ secreetin

D. _____ prostraglandins   I. _____ calsitonen

E. _____ lutinizing   J. _____ trophick

13. Write the meaning of the underlined portion of each word on the line preceding the word.

A. _____ <u>andro</u>gen   F. _____ acromegaly

B. _____ endo<u>crine</u>   G. _____ acromegaly

C. _____ progesterone   H. _____ adrenal

D. _____ pineal   I. _____ adrenal

E. _____ oxytocin   J. _____ <u>para</u>thyroid

14. Using your knowledge of word parts match, the following terms and definitions.

A. _____ Inflammation of the pancreas   A. Adrenalectomy

B. _____ Surgical removal of the pituitary gland   B. Adrenalitis

                                                  C. Endocrinopathy

C. _____ Tumor of the pineal gland   D. Glycosuria

D. _____ Any disorder of the endocrine system   E. Hypophysectomy

E. _____ Surgical removal of an adrenal gland   F. Pancreatalgia

                                                  G. Pancreatitis

F. _____ Inflammation of the adrenal gland   H. Pinealoma

G. _____ Pain in the pancreas   I. Polyphagia

H. _____ Enlargement of the thyroid gland   J. Thyromegaly

I. _____ Presence of glucose in the urine

J. _____ Excessive hunger or eating

15. For each of the following words, underline the word part that corresponds to the underlined word or phrase in the definition.

   A. histamine   a <u>nitrogen compound</u> found in all body tissues

   B. androgens   steroid hormones that promote <u>male</u> characteristics

   C. prolactin   hormone that stimulates production of <u>milk</u>

   D. oxytocin   hormone that stimulates a <u>rapid</u> birth

   E. adrenal   a gland on top of the <u>kidney</u>

   F. polydipsia   excessive <u>thirst</u>

   G. endocrine   glands that <u>secrete</u> their products into the blood

   H. testes   <u>egg</u>-shaped male gonads

   I. gonadotropin   a hormone that <u>influences</u> the gonads

   J. estrogens   steroid hormones that <u>produce</u> female characteristics

TESTING COMPREHENSION

Multiple choice: Select the best response.

1. Of the following pairs of hormones, which pair represents two steroid hormones? (a) insulin and cortisol, (b) aldosterone and epinephrine, (c) insulin and epinephrine, (d) aldosterone and cortisol.

2. Protein hormones (a) utilize cyclic adenosine monophosphate (AMP), (b) include prostaglandins, (c) are relatively slow to respond, (d) bind with receptors inside the cell.

3. Protein hormones are difficult to administer orally because they (a) bind with receptors on the cell membrane, (b) are inactivated in the stomach before they reach target tissue, (c) respond very slowly, (d) use a second messenger system of reaction.

4. An example of a tropic hormone is (a) insulin, (b) epinephrine, (c) TSH, (d) oxytocin.

5. Regulation of secretion by nervous stimulation pertains to (a) epinephrine, (b) insulin, (c) thyroxine, (d) testosterone.

6. The infundibulum of the pituitary gland (a) connects the gland to the sella turcica, (b) attaches the gland to the hypothalamus of the brain, (c) produces tropic hormones, (d) produces oxytocin and ADH.

7. Which of the following hormones are secreted by the adenohypophysis? (a) growth hormone and oxytocin, (b) luteinizing hormone and ADH, (c) prolactin and epinephrine, (d) TSH and adrenocorticotropic hormone.

8. The hormone that is secreted by the neurohypophysis and stimulates the contraction of the pregnant uterus is (a) estrogen, (b) oxytocin, (c) prolactin, (d) luteinizing hormone.

9. The hormone that is secreted by the anterior pituitary gland and stimulates breast development during pregnancy in preparation for lactation is (a) follicle-stimulating hormone, (b) oxytocin, (c) prolactin, (d) growth hormone.

10. Parafollicular cells of the thyroid gland produce (a) triiodothyronine, (b) tetraiodothyronine, (c) thyroxine, (d) calcitonin.

11. Insufficient iodine in the diet results in (a) an increase in active thyroxine, (b) an increase in active calcitonin, (c) an increase in active triiodothyronine, (d) an increase in active TSH.

12. A deficiency of active thyroid hormone in the infant results in (a) cretinism, (b) myxedema, (c) acromegaly, (d) a high metabolic rate.

13. Tetany resulting from low calcium levels in the blood (hypocalcemia) is (a) a result of a deficiency of parathyroid hormone, (b) caused by a calcitonin deficiency, (c) a result of osteoclast activity, (d) caused by a deficiency in activity of follicular cells.

148

14. Hormones from the adrenal cortex are (a) amino acids, (b) prostaglandin, (c) steroids, (d) proteins.

15. Aldosterone is secreted (a) in response to neural stimulation, (b) in response to tropic hormones, (c) in response to sodium and potassium ions, (d) in response to a hormone from the anterior pituitary gland.

16. Two hormones that increase blood glucose levels are (a) cortisol and glucagon, (b) insulin and glucagon, (c) cortisol and insulin, (d) glucagon and melatonin.

17. The pancreas secretes hormones that (a) are concerned with sugar and salt, (b) are controlled by tropic hormones, (c) include both insulin and glucagon, (d) are steroids.

18. The primary function of insulin is to (a) regulate blood volume, (b) stimulate cells to produce glucose, (c) produce an inflammatory response, (d) lower blood glucose levels.

19. The principal androgen is (a) testosterone, (b) interstitial cell stimulating hormone, (c) gonadocorticoid, (d) progesterone.

20. Human chorionic gonadotropin (HCG) is produced by the (a) gastric mucosa, (b) placenta, (c) small intestine, (d) pineal gland.

21. Melatonin is secreted by the (a) pineal gland, (b) thymus gland, (c) gastric mucosa, (d) placenta.

22. Prostaglandins (a) have a widespread effect, (b) are protein hormones, (c) have a long-term effect, (d) are derivations of arachidonic acid.

23. A patient has a tentative diagnosis of hyperthyroidism. What would you expect to observe in the individual? (a) polyuria, (b) insomnia, (c) weight gain, (d) low metabolic rate.

24. Which of the following would you expect to observe in a child with hypopituitarism? (a) hyperpigmentation of the skin, (b) early sexual development, (c) copious dilute urine output, (d) growth failure.

25. Which of the following are associated with the inflammatory response? (a) epinephrine and cortisol, (b) cortisol and prostaglandins, (c) thyroxine and thymosin, (d) prostaglandins and melatonin.

A STEP BEYOND

Go a step beyond the ordinary and learn more about a topic that is related to this chapter but not discussed in detail in the textbook. Select one of the following topics, or one suggested by your instructor, and write a brief paper (250 words minimum), create a poster, or develop a short presentation (approximately 4 to 5 minutes) that focuses on your selection. Suggested topics for this chapter include the following:

1. *Body temperature and the thyroid gland.* What is the relationship of the thyroid gland to body temperature? Investigate this relationship and report your findings.
2. *Diabetes mellitus.* Why do some people with diabetes mellitus have to have insulin injections, but others only take a pill? Compare insulin-dependent diabetes with non–insulin-dependent diabetes, including pathogenesis and treatment. Report your findings.
3. *Chvostek sign.* Ted Annee just had a thyroidectomy. The nurse observed a positive Chvostek sign. What does this mean? Is it a cause for concern? What is the possible relationship between this sign and the thyroidectomy? Report the answers to these questions.
4. *Goiter.* Select a famous person from history who had a simple goiter, and prepare a brief biography of that person.

FUN & GAMES

Word Scramble

Determine the word that fits each definition, and then write the word in the spaces across from the definition, one letter per space. The letters in the boxes form a scrambled word or words. Unscramble the letters to create a word or words that matches the final definition in each section.

1. Secretory product of an endocrine gland

2. Chemical class of lipid soluble hormones

3. Another name for the pituitary gland

4. Another name for lactogenic hormone

5. Central portion of the adrenal gland

Letters to use for final word: _____

Final definition: Any disorder of endocrine glands

_____

6. Principal mineral corticoid

7. A hormone secreted by the ovaries

8. Hormone secreted by the thymus

9. Hormone secreted by the lining of the stomach

10. Gland that secretes melatonin

Letters to use for final word: _____

Final definition: Hormone-like derivatives of arachidonic acid

_____

Cardiovascular System: The Heart

LEARNING EXERCISES

Overview of the Heart

1. All of the following statements are false. Rewrite each statement to make it true.
   A. The base of the heart is directed inferiorly and to the left.

   _____

   B. About a third of the heart mass is on the left side.

   _____

   C. The heart is located in the anterior mediastinum, between the second and fifth ribs.

   _____

2. Arrange the following coverings around the heart in the correct sequence by numbering them in the order in which they occur. Start with 1 for the outermost layer and proceed to 4 for the innermost layer.

   A. _____   Epicardium

   B. _____   Fibrous pericardium

   C. _____   Pericardial cavity

   D. _____   Parietal pericardium

Structure of the Heart

1. Write the terms that best fit the following phrases about the structure of the heart.

   A. _____   Middle layer of the heart wall

   B. _____   Chamber that receives blood from the superior vena cava

   C. _____   Valve between the right atrium and ventricle

   D. _____   Inner lining of the heart wall

   E. _____   Receives oxygenated blood from the lungs

   F. _____   Thin region of the interatrial septum

   G. _____   Receives blood from the right atrium

   H. _____   Ridges of myocardium in the ventricles

   I. _____   Atrioventricular valve on left side of the heart

J. _____ Valve at base of the aorta

K. _____ Arteries that supply blood to the myocardium

L. _____ Chamber that receives blood from the inferior vena cava

2. Trace the pathway of blood through the heart by numbering the following structures in the correct sequence. Start with number 1 for the venae cavae.

A. _____ Aortic semilunar valve   H. _____ Pulmonary trunk

B. _____ Ascending aorta   I. _____ Pulmonary veins

C. _____ Bicuspid valve   J. _____ Pulmonary arteries

D. _____ Capillaries of lungs   K. _____ Right atrium

E. _____ Left atrium   L. _____ Right ventricle

F. _____ Left ventricle   M. _____ Tricuspid valve

G. _____ Pulmonary semilunar valve   N. _____ Venae cavae

Physiology of the Heart

1. Write the terms that best fit the following phrases about the conduction system of the heart and the cardiac cycle.

A. _____ Pacemaker of the heart

B. _____ Length of cardiac cycle at 72 beats/minute

C. _____ Indicates depolarization of the atria on electrocardiography (ECG)

D. _____ Transmits impulses to the atria and atrioventricular (AV) node

E. _____ A recording of the electrical activity of the heart

F. _____ Indicates depolarization of ventricles on ECG

G. _____ Contraction phase of the ventricles

H. _____ Carry impulses to the myocardium

I. _____ Indicates repolarization of the ventricles on ECG

J. _____ Relaxation phase of the ventricles

K. _____ Transmit impulses away from the AV node

L. _____ Length of atrial systole in one cardiac cycle

M. _____ Normally has fastest rate of depolarization

N. _____ Length of ventricular systole in one cycle

2. In the space before each phrase about events in the cardiac cycle, write S if the phrase refers to ventricular systole and write D if it refers to ventricular diastole.

A. _____ Atria are in systole

B. _____ AV valves open

C. _____ AV valves close

D. _____ Semilunar (SL) valves open

E. _____ Semilunar (SL) valves close

F. _____ Blood is ejected from the heart

G. _____ Pressure in ventricles decreases

H. _____ Blood enters the ventricles

3. Heart sounds are associated with heart valves closing. Which valves are associated with the following sounds?

A. First heart sound (lubb)

B. Second heart sound (dupp)

4. In the space before each statement about factors that influence cardiac output, write T if the statement is true and write F if the statement is false. If the statement is false, change the underlined word(s) to make the statement true.

A. _____ Cardiac output equals heart rate plus stroke volume.

B. _____ Stroke volume is the amount of blood ejected from the heart during each cardiac cycle.

C. _____ Increased venous return decreases contraction strength.

D. _____ Sympathetic stimulation decreases contraction strength.

E. _____ Increased contraction strength increases cardiac output.

F. _____ Parasympathetic nerves decrease heart rate.

G. _____ Increased end-diastolic volume decreases stroke volume.

H. _____ Sympathetic stimulation increases heart rate.

I. _____ Increased end-diastolic volume increases cardiac output.

J. _____ Most changes in heart rate are mediated through the cardiac center in the pons.

K. _____ Epinephrine decreases heart rate.

L. _____ Increased carbon dioxide concentration in the tissues increases heart rate.

LABELING AND COLORING EXERCISES

Identify the listed structures of the heart illustrated in Figure 11-1 by matching them with the correct letters from the diagram. Use blue to color the chambers and vessels that contain oxygen-poor blood. Use red to color the chambers and vessels that contain oxygen-rich blood.

1. _____ Right atrium

2. _____ Right ventricle

3. _____ Left atrium

4. _____ Left ventricle

5. _____ Interventricular septum

6. _____ Superior vena cava

7. _____ Inferior vena cava

8. _____ Pulmonary trunk

9. _____ Ascending aorta

10. _____ Right brachiocephalic vein

11. _____ Brachiocephalic artery

12. _____ Aortic semilunar valve

13. _____ Pulmonary semilunar valve

14. _____ Tricuspid valve

15. _____ Bicuspid valve

16. _____ Left common carotid artery

17. _____ Left subclavian artery

18. _____ Left pulmonary artery

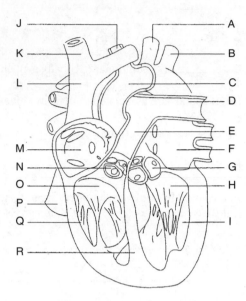

Figure 11-1 Structure of the heart.

19. Figure 11-2 illustrates anterior and posterior views of the heart. Identify the indicated vessels by writing the name of the vessel on the line that corresponds to the letter of the vessel.

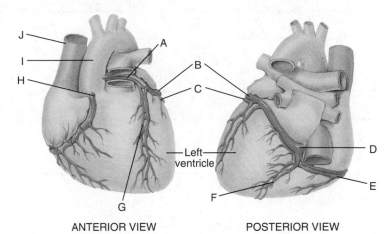

Figure 11-2 Blood supply to the myocardium.

A. _____

B. _____

C. _____

D. _____

E. _____

F. _____

G. _____

H. _____

I. _____

J. _____

20. Figure 11-3 illustrates a segment of an electrocardiogram. Color the P wave red, the QRS complex blue, and the T wave yellow.

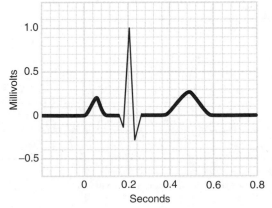

Figure 11-3 Electrocardiogram.

Chapter **11** **Cardiovascular System: The Heart**

1. Specifically where within the middle mediastinum is the heart located? Where is the apex? Where is the base?

_____

_____

2. What are the two main components, or layers, of the pericardial sac?

_____

_____

3. Where is the pericardial cavity?

_____

4. What are the three layers of the heart wall?

_____

_____

_____

5. What is the difference in structure between the atria and ventricles?

_____

_____

6. How does the structural difference in the heart chambers reflect their functional difference?

_____

_____

_____

7. How do atrioventricular valves and semilunar valves differ in structure?

_____

_____

_____

8. How does the structural difference between atrioventricular and semilunar valves reflect their functional difference?

_____

_____

_____

9. Draw a diagram of the heart and identify the chambers and valves.

10. List, in sequence, the structures through which blood passes as it goes from the right atrium to the ascending aorta.

_____

_____

_____

11. How does the myocardium receive the oxygen that is required for contraction?

_____

_____

12. What are the components of the conduction system of the heart? Why is a conduction system necessary?

_____

_____

_____

13. How do the waves, or deflections, of an electrocardiogram relate to events in the conduction system?

_____

_____

_____

14. What is meant by the terms *systole* and *diastole*?

_____

15. What happens during each part of the cardiac cycle, and how long does each part last?

_____

_____

_____

16. How do heart sounds relate to events of the cardiac cycle?

_____

_____

17. How is cardiac output calculated?

_____

18. By what mechanisms does end-diastolic volume affect stroke volume and cardiac output?

_____

_____

_____

19. What center in the brain regulates the rate of the sinoatrial node? Through what pathway does this regulation occur?

_____

_____

FUNCTIONAL RELATIONSHIPS

It is important to remember that no system in the body works alone. It takes the interaction of all systems to maintain homeostasis. The following exercises reinforce the concept that all systems work together to maintain the health and well-being of other systems and the individual.

Match the system on the right with what it provides for the cardiovascular system on the left. Use the functional relationships page in your concepts textbook as a resource.

1. _____ Provides barrier against entry of pathogens

2. _____ Protects heart and thoracic vessels

3. _____ Assists venous return

4. _____ Adjusts heart rate to maintain cardiac output

5. _____ Its products adjust heart rate, contraction strength, blood volume, and blood pressure

6. _____ Fights infections in the heart and returns interstitial fluid to the blood

7. _____ Helps maintain blood pH and provides oxygen for cardiac muscle

8. _____ Absorbs nutrients for blood cell formation

9. _____ Helps maintain blood electrolyte composition

10. _____ Produces hormones that help maintain healthy blood vessels

A. Digestive

B. Endocrine

C. Integumentary

D. Lymphatic

E. Muscular

F. Nervous

G. Reproductive

H. Respiratory

I. Skeletal

J. Urinary

For each of the following systems, write what the cardiovascular system provides for it.

11. Nervous _____

12. Skeletal _____

13. Reproductive_____

14. Endocrine _____

15. Respiratory _____

16. Muscular _____

17. Lymphatic _____

18. Digestive _____

19. Urinary _____

20. Integumentary _____

1. Match the definitions on the left with the correct clinical term from the column on the right by placing the corresponding letter in the space before the definition. Not all terms will be used.

A. _____ Contraction phase of the cardiac cycle

B. _____ Enlargement of the heart

C. _____ Rapid, random, irregular, ineffectual heart contractions

D. _____ Any primary disease of heart muscle

E. _____ Drug that increases strength and regularity of heart contractions

F. _____ Volume of blood ejected from one ventricle during contraction

G. _____ Using a stethoscope to listen to heart sounds

H. _____ Acute chest pain caused by decreased blood supply to heart muscle

I. _____ A vasodilator to relieve the pain of angina pectoris

J. _____ Valves between the heart ventricles and output vessels

1. Angina pectoris
2. Atrioventricular
3. Auscultation
4. Cardiac infarction
5. Cardiac output
6. Cardiomegaly
7. Cardiomyopathy
8. Diastole
9. Digitalis (Digoxin)
10. Fibrillation
11. Nitroglycerin
12. Semilunar
13. Stroke volume
14. Systole

2. Write the meaning of the following abbreviations.

A. _____ CABG

B. _____ PVC

C. _____ CPR

D. _____ VSD

E. _____ CHF

F. _____ CAD

G. _____ LCA

H. _____ ECG

I. _____ MI

J. _____ VT

3. Spelling is important in scientific and medical applications because only one or two incorrect letters can change the meaning. All of the following words are from this chapter and are spelled incorrectly. Write the correct spelling in the space preceding the misspelled words.

A. _____ arhythmia

B. _____ infarcshun

C. _____ distole

D. _____ conjestive

E. _____ fosa ovalis

F. _____ interkallaated

G. _____ sistolee

H. _____ atreum

I. _____ pappilary

J. _____ semiloonar

4. Write the meaning of the underlined portion of each word on the line preceding the word.

A. _____ epicardium

B. _____ myocardium

C. _____ stenosis

D. _____ tachycardia

E. _____ electrocardiogram

F. _____ semilunar

G. _____ sphygmomanometer

H. _____ coronary

I. _____ echocardiogram

J. _____ stethoscope

5. Complete the following terms for the given definitions.

A. Disease condition of heart muscle   cardio_____

B. Condition of rapid heartbeat   _____cardia

C. Narrowing of the mitral valve   mitral_____

D. Pertaining to an upper heart chamber   _____al

E. Surgical repair of a valve   valvulo_____

F. Condition of slow heartbeat   _____cardia

G. Enlargement of the heart   cardio_____

H. Wall between the right and left atria of the heart   atrial_____

I. Instrument for recording the energy of a pulse   sphygmo _____

J. Surgical puncture into the pericardial
   cavity with aspiration of fluid   pericardio _____

6. For each of the following words, underline the word part that corresponds to the underlined word or phrase in the definition.

A. bradycardia	<u>slow</u> heart rate	F. tachycardia	rapid <u>heart</u> rate
B. semilunar	half-<u>moon</u> shaped	G. cardiomegaly	<u>enlargement</u> of the heart
C. ultrasonography	records <u>sound</u> waves	H. tricuspid	heart valve with three <u>points</u>
D. mitral stenosis	<u>narrowing</u> of left AV valve	I. atrium	<u>entrance chamber</u> of the heart
E. sphygmomanometer	instrument for recording <u>pulse</u>	J. stethoscope	instrument used to hear sound in the <u>chest</u>

TESTING COMPREHENSION

Multiple choice: Select the best response.

1. In normal position, the apex of the heart is directed (a) inferiorly and to the left, (b) superiorly and to the left, (c) inferiorly and to the right, (d) superiorly and to the right.

2. The heart is located in the (a) anterior mediastinum, (b) middle mediastinum, (c) superior mediastinum, (d) posterior mediastinum.

3. The lining of the pericardial sac is a layer of (a) parietal mucous membrane, (b) visceral mucosa membrane, (c) parietal serous membrane, (d) visceral serous membrane.

4. The outermost layer of the heart wall is (a) a parietal serous membrane, (b) a visceral mucous membrane, (c) the endocardium, (d) a visceral serous membrane.

5. The muscle in the heart wall (a) has spindle-shaped fibers with tapered ends, (b) is voluntary muscle, (c) is nonstriated, (d) has intercalated disks.

6. Most of the heart wall is (a) pericardium, (b) myocardium, (c) endocardium, (d) epicardium.

7. The chamber of the heart that receives blood from the superior vena cava is the (a) right atrium, (b) left atrium, (c) right ventricle, (d) left ventricle.

8. The two chambers of the heart that contain oxygen poor blood are the (a) right atrium and left atrium, (b) right ventricle and left ventricle, (c) right atrium and right ventricle, (d) left atrium and left ventricle.

9. The chambers of the heart that have papillary muscle are the (a) right atrium and left atrium, (b) right ventricle and left ventricle, (c) right atrium and right ventricle, (d) left atrium and left ventricle.

10. The bicuspid valve is between the (a) right atrium and left atrium, (b) right ventricle and left ventricle, (c) right atrium and right ventricle, (d) left atrium and left ventricle.

11. The chamber of the heart that pumps blood into the pulmonary trunk is the (a) right atrium, (b) right ventricle, (c) left atrium, (d) left ventricle.

12. The portion of the conduction system of the heart that sets the normal rhythm of the heart beat is the (a) SA node, (b) AV node, (c) bundle branch, (d) conduction myofibers.

13. The portion of the conduction system of the heart that delays the impulse prior to ventricular contraction is the (a) SA node, (b) AV node, (c) bundle branch, (d) conduction myofibers.

14. In a normal cardiac cycle, atrial systole last for about (a) 0.1 second, (b) 0.3 second, (c) 0.4 second, (d) 0.7 second.

15. Blood is ejected from the heart during (a) atrial systole, (b) atrial diastole, (c) ventricular systole, (d) ventricular diastole.

16. What normally prevents blood from flowing back into the ventricle from the aorta? (a) pulmonary semilunar valve, (b) tricuspid valve, (c) bicuspid valve, (d) aortic semilunar valve.

17. The artery in the left atrioventricular sulcus is the (a) marginal artery, (b) circumflex artery, (c) anterior descending coronary artery, (d) left coronary artery.

18. The quantity of blood that is ejected from the left ventricle during one cardiac cycle is the (a) cardiac output, (b) end diastolic volume, (c) stroke volume, (d) end systolic volume.

19. The portion of an ECG that records the electrical activity during atrial systole is the (a) P wave, (b) Q wave, (c) QRS complex, (d) T wave.

20. About 70% of ventricular filling occurs during the time when (a) the atria are in systole, (b) the ventricles are in systole, (c) atria are in systole and the ventricles are in diastole, (d) the atria and ventricles are in diastole.

21. Which of the following is *least* likely to increase cardiac output? (a) increased stimulation by the vagus nerve, (b) increased venous return, (c) increased stroke volume, (d) increased heart rate.

22. An increase in the volume of ventricular filling (a) stimulates the vagus nerve, (b) increases stroke volume, (c) closes the AV valves, (d) increases coronary blood flow.

23. Left-sided heart failure resulting from a myocardial infarction is likely to cause (a) an increase in parasympathetic stimulation, (b) an increase in venous return, (c) an increase in stroke volume, (d) an accumulation of blood in the pulmonary veins.

24. The physician prescribed nitroglycerin for a patient with angina pectoris. The desired effect of this medication is to (a) improve coronary blood flow, (b) constrict peripheral blood vessels, (c) increase contraction strength of the heart, (d) increase heart rate.

25. Mr. Cory Nairee went to his physician for a routine check-up. The physician detected a heart murmur. Heart murmurs are caused by (a) an enlarged heart, (b) congestive heart failure, (c) pericarditis, (d) faulty heart valves.

A STEP BEYOND

Go a step beyond the ordinary and learn more about a topic that is related to this chapter but not discussed in detail in the textbook. Select one of the following topics, or one suggested by your instructor, and write a brief paper (250 words minimum), create a poster, or develop a short presentation (approximately 4 to 5 minutes) that focuses on your selection. Suggested topics for this chapter include the following:

1. *First human heart transplant.* Who performed the first human heart transplant? When? Where? What was the outcome, i.e., how long did the patient live following the procedure?
2. *Cardiac therapy.* Several different therapies are used to assist or control the function of the heart. Define and illustrate the inotropic effects, chronotropic effects, and dromotropic effects of cardiac treatments and/or therapies.
3. *Heart failure.* Compare the signs, symptoms, and treatment of right-sided heart failure with those of left-sided heart failure.
4. *Cardiac drugs.* The autonomic nervous system has an important role in regulating heart rate and contraction strength. Therapeutic drugs for the heart may be classified by the way in which they affect the autonomic nervous system receptors. Define *beta-adrenergic receptors* and *muscarinic receptors*. Give examples of drugs that activate and block each type of receptor and the effect they have on the heart.

Word Scramble

Determine the word that fits each definition, and then write the word in the spaces across from the definition, one letter per space. The letters in the boxes form a scrambled word or words. Unscramble the letters to create a word or words that matches the final definition in each section.

1. Necrosis of muscle due to lack of oxygen

2. End of the heart opposite the apex

3. Pumping chamber of the heart

4. Another name for bicuspid valve

Letters to use for final word: _____

Final definition: Rapid, random, irregular contractions of the heart

_____

5. Lining of the heart wall

6. Muscular layer of the heart wall

7. Chamber that receives blood from the inferior vena cava

8. Any primary disease of heart muscle

Letters to use for final word: _____

Final definition: Noninvasive cardiac procedure that uses sound waves

_____

12 Cardiovascular System: The Blood Vessels

LEARNING EXERCISES

Classification and Structure of Blood Vessels

1. Indicate whether each of the following refers to an artery (A), a capillary (C), or a vein (V).

A. _____ Carries blood away from the heart

B. _____ Functions in the exchange of substances between blood and tissue cells

C. _____ Wall consists of simple squamous epithelium

D. _____ Carries blood toward the heart

E. _____ Has valves

F. _____ Has three relatively thick layers in the wall

G. _____ Has three relatively thin layers in the wall

H. _____ May have vasa vasorum

2. Name the tunic or layer in the wall of a blood vessel that contains predominately

A. connective tissue _____

B. simple squamous epithelium _____

C. smooth muscle _____

Physiology of Circulation

1. Identify the passive transport process by which each of the following substances moves through the capillary wall.

A. _____ Carbon dioxide

B. _____ Oxygen

C. _____ Water (2)

_____

2. Write an *A* before the phrases that pertain to the arterial end of a capillary and a *V* before the phrases that pertain to the venule end of a capillary.

A. _____ Osmotic pressure is greater than hydrostatic pressure

B. _____ Hydrostatic pressure is greater than osmotic pressure

C. _____ Net movement of fluid out of the capillary

D. _____ Net movement of fluid into the capillary

3. In the spaces on the left, write the answers that match the statements about blood flow and blood pressure.

A. _____ Vessel with the greatest pressure

B. _____ Type of vessel with greatest area

C. _____ Type of vessel with the lowest pressure

D. _____ Type of vessel with the slowest blood flow

E. _____ Vessel with the fastest blood flow

F. _____ Primary force that moves blood

G. _____ Actions that move blood through veins (3)

_____

_____

H. _____ Pressure during ventricular contraction

I. _____ Pressure during ventricular relaxation

J. _____ Instrument used to measure blood pressure

K. _____ Systolic pressure minus diastolic pressure

L. _____ Blood flow sounds heard in a stethoscope

M. _____ Effect of increased CO_2 on precapillary sphincters

4. Indicate whether each of the following will increase (I) or decrease (D) the rate of blood flow to a specific area.

A. _____ Increase in blood pressure

B. _____ Increase in resistance

C. _____ Increase in cardiac output

D. _____ Vasodilation

E. _____ Increase in carbon dioxide concentration

F. _____ Contraction of precapillary sphincters

G. _____ Decrease in pH

5. Indicate whether each of the following refers to systolic pressure (S), diastolic pressure (D), or pulse pressure (P).

A. _____ Pressure at which the first Korotkoff sound is heard

B. _____ Normal is about 40 mm Hg

C. _____ Blood begins to flow freely through the arteries

D. _____ Normal is about 120 mm Hg

E. _____ Normal is about 80 mm Hg

Chapter 12 Cardiovascular System: The Blood Vessels

6. In the spaces on the left, write answers that match the statements about the regulation of blood pressure.

A. _____ Location of vasomotor and cardiac centers

B. _____ Center that regulates heart rate

C. _____ Center that regulates blood vessel diameter

D. _____ Type of receptors that respond when vessel walls stretch

E. _____ Type of receptors that respond to carbon dioxide and hydrogen ion concentrations

F. _____ Substance produced by the kidneys that has a role in blood pressure regulation

G. _____ Actions of angiotensin that increase blood pressure (2)

   _____

H. _____ Hormone that conserves sodium ions to increase blood pressure

7. Place a check (√) in the appropriate column to indicate whether the given condition tends to increase or decrease blood pressure

Given Condition	Increase	Decrease
A marked increase in blood volume		
An increase in heart rate		
Polycythemia		
Loss of body fluids		
Sympathetic stimulation of arterioles		
Production of angiotensin		
Slow heartbeat		

CIRCULATORY PATHWAYS

1. In the space at the left, write the name of the artery that is described.

A. _____ Branches from the ascending aorta

B. _____ First, or most anterior, branch of aortic arch

C. _____ Branch of the aortic arch to the left arm

D. _____ Paired vessels that go to the brain (2)

   _____

E. _____ Middle branch of the aortic arch

2. Name the major arteries described by each phrase.

A. _____ Located in the arm

B. _____ Located on the lateral side of the forearm

C. _____ Located on the medial side of the forearm

D. _____ Branch of celiac that supplies the liver

E. _____ Branch of celiac that supplies the stomach

F. _____ Supplies the pancreas and spleen

G. _____ Supplies the small intestine and part of the colon

H. _____ Paired vessels to the kidneys

I. _____ Supplies the descending colon and rectum

J. _____ Formed by bifurcation of the aorta

K. _____ Enters the pelvis and supplies the urinary bladder

L. _____ Located in the thigh region

M. _____ Located in the posterior knee region

N. _____ Supplies the posterior portion of the leg

O. _____ Supplies the anterior portion of the leg

3. Name the major veins described by each phrase.

A. _____ Large veins that enter the right atrium (2)

B. _____

C. _____ Join to form the superior vena cava

D. _____ Major vein from the brain

E. _____ Superficial vein on the medial side of the arm

F. _____ Superficial vein on the lateral side of the arm

G. _____ Vein at the elbow used for drawing blood

H. _____ Deep vein in the arm

I. _____ Drains the muscle tissue of the abdominal wall

J. _____ Vein from the liver that enters the inferior vena cava

Chapter **12** **Cardiovascular System: The Blood Vessels**

K. _____ Vein that carries nutrient-rich blood to the liver

L. _____ Veins that form the hepatic portal vein (2)

_____

M. _____ Longest vein in the body

N. _____ Join to form the inferior vena cava

O. _____ Drains blood from the pelvic viscera

P. _____ Large deep vein in the thigh

Q. _____ Drains the dorsal foot and anterior leg muscles

R. _____ Drains the posterior leg muscles

4. Name the feature of fetal circulation described by each phrase.

A. _____ Transports blood from the fetus to the placenta

B. _____ Transports blood from the placenta to the fetus

C. _____ Bypasses the liver

D. _____ Opening in the interatrial septum

E. _____ Shunt from the pulmonary trunk to the aorta

F. _____ Structure where gaseous exchange occurs

5. Fill in the blanks with the correct blood vessels and valves to complete the pathway of pulmonary circulation.

A. right atrium

B. _____

C. right ventricle

D. _____

E. _____

F. _____

G. capillaries of lungs

H. _____

I. left atrium

6. Follow the pathway for the flow of blood from the left ventricle to the right middle cerebral artery by filling in the blanks.

A. left ventricle

B. aortic semilunar valve

C. _____

D. aortic arch

E. _____

F. _____

G. _____

H. right middle cerebral artery

7. Follow the pathway for the flow of blood from the left gonad (ovary or testicle) to the lateral side of the left forearm by filling in the blanks.

A. left gonad

B. left gonadal vein

C. _____

D. _____

E. _____

F. _____ valve

G. _____

H. _____ valve

I. _____

J. _____

K. capillaries of lungs

L. _____

M. _____

N. _____ valve

O. _____

P. _____ valve

Q. _____

R. aortic arch

S. _____

T. _____

U. _____

V. _____

W. capillaries on lateral side of left forearm

8. Follow the pathway for the flow of blood from the descending aorta to the capillaries of the spleen and then to the right atrium by filling in the blanks.

A. descending aorta

B. _____

C. _____

D. capillaries of the spleen

E. _____

F. _____

G. sinusoids of the liver

H. _____

I. _____

J. right atrium

LABELING AND COLORING EXERCISES

1. Figure 12-1 represents the scheme of circulation in the body. Color the portions that contain oxygenated blood red, and color the portions that contain oxygen-poor blood blue. Label the chambers of the heart, pulmonary arteries, pulmonary veins, systemic arteries, and systemic veins as indicated.

A. _____

B. _____

C. _____

D. _____

E. _____

F. _____

G. _____

H. _____

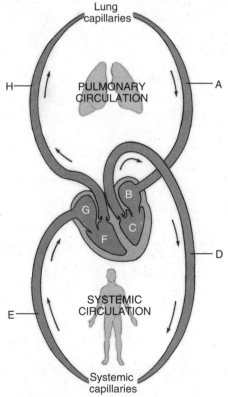

Figure 12-1 Scheme of circulation.

2. Identify the pulse points indicated on Figure 12-2.

A. _____

B. _____

C. _____

D. _____

E. _____

F. _____

G. _____

H. _____

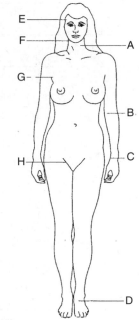

Figure 12-2 Pulse points.

3. Identify the arteries at the base of the brain as indicated on Figure 12-3.

A. _____

B. _____

C. _____

D. _____

E. _____

F. _____

G. _____

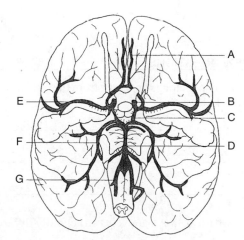

Figure 12-3 Arterial supply to the brain.

171

4. Identify the veins of the hepatic portal system as indicated on Figure 12-4.

A. _____

B. _____

C. _____

D. _____

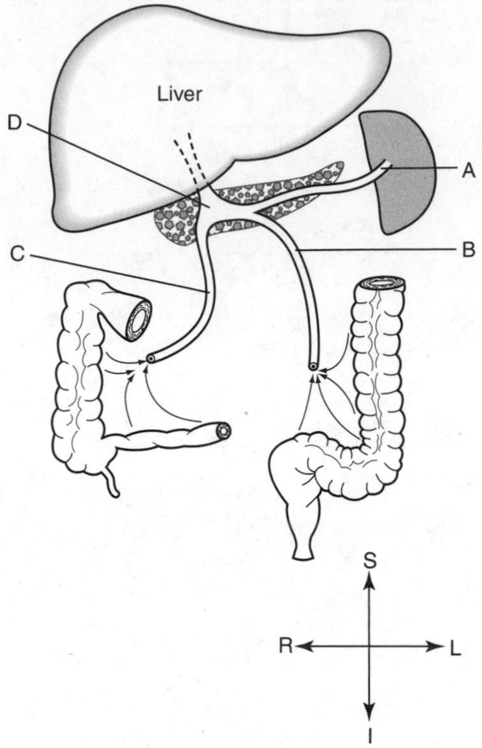

Figure 12-4 Hepatic portal system.

REVIEW QUESTIONS

1. If a pin penetrates an artery from the outside into the lumen, name the layers of the arterial wall, in sequence, through which it passes.

_____

_____

_____

2. In what two ways are veins structurally different from arteries?

_____

_____

3. By what transport mechanism do oxygen and carbon dioxide move across the capillary wall?

_____

4. What two pressures determine fluid movement across the capillary wall?

_____

5. As blood flows from the aorta into the more numerous smaller vessels, what happens to the rate of flow?

_____

_____

6. Why does blood tend to pool, or accumulate, in the legs and feet when a person stands in one place for a long period?

_____

_____

7. What superficial artery in the wrist is used to take the pulse?

_____

8. If you are given the information that the diastolic pressure is 78 mm Hg and the systolic pressure is 115 mm Hg, what is the pulse pressure?

_____

9. When blood vessels lose their elasticity as a result of aging or atherosclerosis, what happens to the blood pressure?

_____

_____

10. Suppose baroreceptors in the aortic arch detect a sudden increase in blood pressure and generate action potentials. What part of the brain receives these action potentials, and how does it respond?

_____

_____

_____

11. The kidneys secrete renin in response to decreases in blood pressure. By what mechanism does renin cause an increase in the blood pressure?

_____

_____

_____

12. Through what two valves does the blood pass to get from the right atrium to the lungs to receive a new supply of oxygen?

_____

13. What branch of the aortic arch supplies blood to the right arm and the right side of the head and neck?

_____

14. What branch of the subclavian artery ascends the neck to supply blood to the brain?

_____

15. What two vessels join to form the superior vena cava?

_____

16. Trace the path of blood from the abdominal aorta to the spleen and back to the inferior vena cava.

A. _____   D. _____   G. _____

B. _____   E. _____   H. _____

C. _____   F. _____   I. _____

17. What two features of the circulatory pathway in the fetus allow blood to bypass the immature lungs?

_____

_____

_____

VOCABULARY PRACTICE

1. Match the definitions on the left with the correct clinical term from the column on the right by placing the corresponding letter in the space before the definition. Not all terms will be used.

A. _____ Sounds heard in the stethoscope when taking blood pressure

B. _____ Increase in size of the lumen of blood vessels

C. _____ A calcium-channel blocker that may be used in the treatment of hypertension

D. _____ Varicose veins in the anal canal

E. _____ Inflammation of veins

F. _____ Opposition to blood flow

G. _____ A diuretic used to decrease blood pressure

H. _____ Surgical repair of a blood vessel

I. _____ A benign tumor of a blood vessel

J. _____ Deficiency in blood supply due to constriction or obstruction of a vessel

1. Angioplasty
2. Arterectomy
3. Diltiazem hydrochloride
4. Furosemide
5. Hemangioma
6. Hemorrhoids
7. Ischemia
8. Korotkoff
9. Peripheral resistance
10. Phlebitis
11. Vasoconstriction
12. Vasodilation

2. Write the meaning of the following abbreviations.

A. _____ CVP   F. _____ PVD

B. _____ DSA   G. _____ DVT

C. _____ ABP   H. _____ SMA

D. _____ PTCA   I. _____ IVC

E. _____ H&H   J. _____ TEE

3. Spelling is important in scientific and medical applications because only one or two incorrect letters can change the meaning. All of the following words are from this chapter and are spelled incorrectly. Write the correct spelling in the space preceding the misspelled words.

A. _____ sfincters   F. _____ flebitis

B. _____ distolic   G. _____ ileac

C. _____ sphygmanometer H. _____ mesentaric

D. _____ peracardial   I. _____ brakioccfalic

E. _____ aneurism   J. _____ safenus

4. Write the meaning of the underlined portion of each word on the line preceding the word.

A. _____ <u>athero</u>sclerosis   F. _____ arterio<u>stenosis</u>

B. _____ is<u>chem</u>ia   G. _____ athero<u>scler</u>osis

C. _____ <u>brachi</u>ocephalic   H. _____ brachio<u>cephal</u>ic

D. _____ arterio<u>ven</u>ous   I. _____ <u>phleb</u>itis

E. _____ <u>vas</u>orum   J. _____ <u>thromb</u>angiitis

5. Use these word parts to write clinical terms that fit the given definitions.

angi-   dermat-   -itis   thrombo-
arter-   -ectomy   phleb-

A. _____   Inflammation of blood vessels in the skin

B. _____   Surgical excision of a vein

C. _____   Inflammation of any blood vessel

D. _____   Surgical excision of an artery

E. _____   Inflammation of a vein associated with clot formation

175

6. For each of the following words, underline the word part that corresponds to the underlined word or phrase in the definition.

   A. aneurysm   local dilation or <u>widening</u> of an arterial wall

   B. angiorraphy   suture of a blood <u>vessel</u>

   C. ischemia   <u>deficiency</u> of blood supply to a region

   D. thrombongiitis   inflammation of a blood vessel with the formation of a <u>clot</u>

   E. arteriosclerosis   <u>hardening</u> of an artery

   F. atherogenesis   formation of <u>fatty plaques</u> in the wall of an artery

   G. angiorraphy   <u>suture</u> of a blood vessel

   H. thrombongiitis   inflammation of a <u>blood vessel</u> with the formation of a clot

   I. atherogenesis   <u>formation</u> of fatty plaques in the wall of an artery

   J. ischemia   <u>condition</u> resulting from a deficiency of <u>blood</u> supply to a region

TESTING COMPREHENSION

Multiple choice: Select the best response.

1. The middle layer of an arterial wall is (a) simple squamous epithelium, (b) smooth muscle, (c) connective tissue, (d) elastic cartilage.

2. One of the differences between veins and arteries is that (a) veins have two layers in the wall and arteries have three layers; (b) the tunica intima in veins is simple squamous epithelium, and in arteries it is stratified squamous epithelium; (c) veins have thinner walls than arteries; (d) veins have more smooth muscle than arteries.

3. Which of the following is *not* true about capillaries? (a) the tunica externa, tunica media, and tunica intima are present but very thin; (b) capillaries have a large total cross-sectional area; (c) blood flow into a capillary bed is controlled by precapillary sphincters; (d) the thin capillary walls permit exchange of materials between the blood and tissue cells.

4. When a precapillary sphincter contracts, (a) blood is forced into the capillaries, (b) blood flows through metarterioles into veins, (c) blood backs up in the arteries, (d) the rate of blood flow slows to allow more time for diffusion.

5. At any given time, approximately what percentage of blood volume is in the systemic veins? (a) 5%, (b) 10%, (c) 40%, (d) 70%.

6. Substances pass through capillary walls by (a) pinocytosis, filtration, and active transport; (b) osmosis and phagocytosis; (c) diffusion and active transport; (d) diffusion, osmosis, and filtration.

7. At the arteriole end of a capillary, water moves from the plasma into the interstitial fluid by (a) filtration, (b) osmosis, (c) diffusion, (d) active transport.

8. At the arteriole end of a capillary, oxygen and glucose leave the plasma and enter the interstitial fluid by (a) filtration, (b) osmosis, (c) diffusion, (d) active transport.

9. Most of the water that enters the interstitial fluid at the arteriole end of the capillary returns to the blood at the venous end. The transport process at the venous end is (a) filtration, (b) osmosis, (c) diffusion, (d) active transport.

10. Central venous pressure is the blood pressure in the (a) right atrium, (b) femoral vein, (c) descending aorta, (d) left atrium.

11. The rate of blood flow is greatest in the (a) aorta, (b) superior vena cava, (c) femoral artery, (d) brachial artery.

12. The rate of blood flow is slowest in the (a) aorta, (b) inferior vena cava, (c) capillaries, (d) femoral vein.

13. Blood flow in the veins is enhanced by (a) increased resistance, (b) increased skeletal muscle action, (c) decreased hydrostatic pressure, (d) decreased respiratory movements.

14. If systolic pressure is 118 mm Hg and diastolic pressure is 82 mm Hg, then pulse pressure is (a) 200 mm Hg, (b) 40 mm Hg, (c) 100 mm Hg, (d) 36 mm Hg.

15. The pressure at which the first Korotkoff sound is heard is the (a) pulse pressure, (b) diastolic pressure, (c) systolic pressure, (d) venous pressure.

16. When peripheral resistance increases, (a) blood volume increases, (b) viscosity of the blood increases, (c) cardiac output increases, (d) blood pressure increases.

17. During exercise, sympathetic impulses cause (a) dilation of blood vessels in the skin, (b) dilation of blood vessels in the skeletal muscles, (c) dilation of blood vessels in the viscera, (d) dilation of precapillary sphincters in the skin.

18. Angiotensin increases blood pressure by (a) causing vasoconstriction, (b) increasing cardiac output, (c) increasing blood volume, (d) increasing parasympathetic stimulation.

19. The enzyme that is produced by the kidneys and has an influence on blood pressure is (a) angiotensin, (b) aldosterone, (c) renin, (d) secretin.

20. Oxygen-poor blood is found in the (a) pulmonary artery, (b) coronary artery, (c) splenic artery, (d) hepatic artery.

21. The vessels that arise from the ascending aorta are the (a) right and left subclavian arteries, (b) right and left brachiocephalic arteries, (c) right and left coronary arteries, (d) right and left common carotid arteries.

22. The major arteries that supply oxygenated blood to the brain are the (a) external and internal carotid arteries, (b) internal carotid and vertebral arteries, (c) external carotid and vertebral arteries, (d) vertebral artery and middle cerebral artery.

23. Blood from the celiac trunk flows into the (a) superior mesenteric artery, (b) renal artery, (c) common iliac artery, (d) splenic artery.

24. Venous blood from the large intestine first enters the (a) splenic vein, (b) inferior mesenteric vein, (c) hepatic portal vein, (d) superior mesenteric vein.

25. The superior vena cava is formed by the (a) right and left common carotid veins, (b) right and left internal jugular veins, (c) the right and left brachiocephalic veins, (d) the right and left subclavian veins.

A STEP BEYOND

Go a step beyond the ordinary and learn more about a topic that is related to this chapter but not discussed in detail in the textbook. Select one of the following topics, or one suggested by your instructor, and write a brief paper (250 words minimum), create a poster, or develop a short presentation (approximately 4 to 5 minutes) that focuses on your selection. Suggested topics for this chapter include the following:

1. Many people develop varicose veins. Describe the population segments at risk, the cause, pathogenesis, potential complications, and treatment of varicose veins.
2. What is phlebitis? How and why does it develop? What complications can occur, and what can be done to treat phlebitis?
3. Mr. Hy Pertensey routinely has systolic pressure readings of 160 to 170 mm Hg. His diastolic readings are also elevated. In addition to prescribing a pharmaceutical preparation, his physician recommends that he regularly exercise at least 30 minutes a day. Why? What is the relationship of exercise to blood pressure?
4. What is deep vein thrombosis, and where in the body is it most likely to occur. What precautions can be taken to avoid it? What complications may occur? What is an IVC (inferior vena cava) filter, and when is it used?
5. You may frequently hear the terms *stent* and *angioplasty*. Both refer to surgical procedures on blood vessels. Define the two terms and explain the differences in them. What is the most common use of these procedures?

FUN & GAMES

Word Scramble

Determine the word that fits each definition, and then write the word in the spaces across from the definition, one letter per space. The letters in the boxes form a scrambled word or words. Unscramble the letters to create a word (or words) matching the final definition in each section.

1. Vessels that return blood to the heart

2. Narrowing of blood vessels

3. Innermost layer of an arterial wall

Letters to use for final words: _____

Final definition: Blood vessels of the blood vessels

_____

4. Inflammation of veins

5. Smallest blood vessels

6. Enzyme secreted by the kidneys

7. Largest artery in the body

8. Physical property of blood that affects blood pressure

Letters to use for final word: _____

Final definition: Characterized by the buildup of fatty plaques in the wall of vessels

_____

13 Cardiovascular System: Blood

Functions and Characteristics of Blood

1. Write the terms that best fit the following phrases about the functions and characteristics of blood.

A. _____ pH range of the blood

B. _____ Normal volume of blood

C. _____ Types of substances transported by blood (3)

_____

_____

D. _____ Regulatory functions of blood (3)

_____

_____

Composition of Blood

1. The following statement is false. Rewrite the statement to make it true. Blood is 70% plasma and 30% formed elements.

_____

_____

2. Complete the following table about plasma proteins.

Plasma Protein	Percent of Total	Function
	60%	
Globulin		
		Blood clotting

3. Give two examples for each of the following plasma components.

Nonprotein molecules that contain nitrogen   Gases

A. _____   C. _____

_____   _____

Nutrients   Electrolytes

B. _____   D. _____

_____   _____

4. Write the scientific term for each of the three types of formed elements in the blood.

   A. Red blood cells (RBCs)   _____

   B. White blood cells (WBCs) _____

   C. Platelets   _____

5. Write the terms that best fit the following phrases about the formed elements of blood.

   A. _____   Anucleate biconcave disks

   B. _____   Immature RBCs circulating in the blood

   C. _____   Normal range of RBCs/mm³ in blood

   D. _____   Large protein pigment in RBCs

   E. _____   Process by which WBCs enter tissue spaces

   F. _____   Normal range of WBCs/mm³ in blood

   G. _____   Most numerous leukocyte

   H. _____   Leukocyte with red-staining granules

   I. _____   Contains histamine and heparin

   J. _____   Largest leukocyte

   K. _____   Function in antibody production

   L. _____   Multilobed nucleus

   M. _____   Called macrophages in the tissues

   N. _____   Phagocytic granulocyte

   O. _____   Phagocytic agranulocyte

   P. _____   Called mast cells in the tissues

   Q. _____   Help counteract effects of histamine

   R. _____   Function of thrombocytes

   S. _____   Normal range of platelets/mm³ in the blood

   T. _____   Cell that breaks apart to form platelets

6. Indicate whether each of the following pertains to erythrocytes (E), leukocytes (L), or thrombocytes (T).

A. _____ Fragments of large cells

B. _____ Contain hemoglobin

C. _____ May have granules in the cytoplasm

D. _____ Some are phagocytic

E. _____ Biconcave disks

F. _____ Platelets

G. _____ Transport oxygen

H. _____ Primary function is blood clotting

I. _____ Function in prevention of disease

J. _____ Normal number is about 5 million/mm^3

7. Write the terms that best fit the following phrases about erythrocyte productions.

A. _____ Stem cell in the bone marrow

B. _____ Hormone that stimulates RBC production

C. _____ Mineral necessary for healthy RBCs

D. _____ Vitamins necessary for RBC production (2)

_____

E. _____ Necessary for absorption of vitamin B$_{12}$

F. _____ Average life span of RBCs

G. _____ Organs where old RBCs are phagocytized (2)

_____

H. _____ Waste product of RBC destruction

Hemostasis

1. Write the terms that best fit the following phrases about hemostasis.

A. _____ Initial reaction in hemostasis

B. _____ Process of collagen attracting platelets

C. _____ Vitamin necessary for clot formation

D. _____ Mineral necessary for clot formation

E. _____ Dissolution of a clot

2. Number the following events of hemostasis in the sequence in which they occur. The first event is 1, and the final event is 5.

A. _____ Prothrombin is converted to thrombin

B. _____ Smooth muscle in vessel walls contracts

C. _____ Formation of prothrombin activator

D. _____ Fibrinogen is converted to fibrin

E. _____ Collagen attracts platelets to form platelet plug

3. The formation of a blood clot is a complex series of chemical reactions that require numerous clotting factors that are in the platelets. These reactions can be summarized in three stages.

   Stage 1: Damaged tissues release factors that result in the formation of substance A.
   Stage 2: Substance A reacts with ions B to convert substance C into substance D.
   Stage 3: Substance D reacts with ions E to convert substance F into substance G.

   Substance G is the foundation of the clot. What are the reactants and products in these three stages?

   A. Substance A   _____

   B. Ions E   _____

   C. Ions B   _____

   D. Substance F   _____

   E. Substance C   _____

   F. Substance G   _____

   G. Substance D   _____

Blood Typing and Transfusions

1. Complete the following table about the different ABO blood types. For the permissible donor column, assume that a person with the given blood type needs a transfusion and the preferred type is not available. What are the other possible donor types? For the permissible recipient column, what blood types may receive the indicated type if the preferred type is not available?

Blood Type	Agglutinogen	Agglutinin	Permissible Donors	Permissible Recipients
A				
	B			
		None		
	None			

2. Indicate whether each of the following pertains to blood type A, B, AB, or O. Some may have more than one answer.

   A. _____   Has anti-A agglutinins

   B. _____   Can be given to type B individuals

   C. _____   Has no agglutinogens

   D. _____   Universal recipient

   E. _____   Has no agglutinins

   F. _____   Can be given to type O individuals

   G. _____   Can donate to type A individuals

   H. _____   Has type B agglutinogens

I. _____ Universal donor

J. _____ Reacts with type AB donor blood

3. Write the terms that best fit the following phrases about Rh+ and Rh− blood.

   A. _____ Agglutinogen in Rh+ blood

   B. _____ Agglutinogen in Rh− blood

   C. _____ Agglutinin in unsensitized Rh+ blood

   D. _____ Agglutinin in unsensitized Rh− blood

4. Answer the following questions about Rh+ and Rh− blood.

   A. What happens if an unsensitized Rh− individual receives Rh+ blood?

   _____

   B. What happens if a sensitized Rh− individual receives Rh+ blood?

   _____

   C. An Rh+ individual does not develop anti-Rh antibodies after receiving Rh− blood. Why?

   _____

   D. What maternal and fetal blood types may lead to hemolytic disease of the newborn?

   Maternal type: _____   Fetal type: _____

5. Indicate whether each of the following statements is true (T) or false (F).

   A. _____ When Rh− blood is given to an Rh+ individual, the Rh+ individual develops anti-Rh agglutinins.

   B. _____ When Rh+ blood is given to an Rh− individual, the Rh− individual develops anti-Rh agglutinogens.

   C. _____ Hemolytic disease of the newborn may develop when the mother is Rh− and the fetus is Rh+.

   D. _____ Hemolytic disease of the newborn causes agglutination and hemolysis of the fetal blood.

   E. _____ If hemolytic disease of the newborn develops, the fetus should receive a transfusion of Rh+ blood.

LABELING AND COLORING EXERCISES

1. Identify each of the formed elements illustrated in Figure 13-1 by matching the letters with the names. Color the granulocytes yellow and color the agranulocytes green.

   A. _____ Basophil

   B. _____ Eosinophil

   C. _____ Erythrocyte

   D. _____ Lymphocyte

   E. _____ Monocyte

   F. _____ Neutrophil

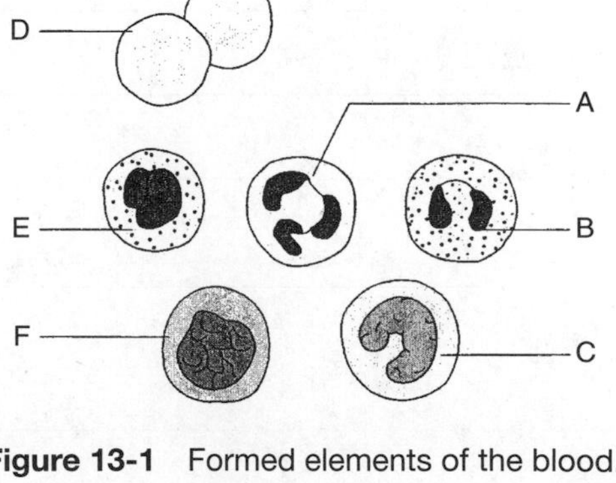

Figure 13-1 Formed elements of the blood.

Chapter **13** **Cardiovascular System: Blood**

2. Figure 13-2 represents a test tube of blood that has been centrifuged to separate the components. Color the plasma portion yellow, and color the erythrocyte portion red. Leave the portion that represents leukocytes and platelets uncolored. Indicate the normal percentage values for A and B.

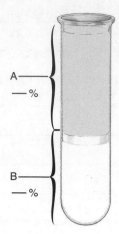

A —— ——%

B —— ——%

Figure 13-2   Composition of blood.

REVIEW QUESTIONS

1. What is the total volume of blood in the human body? What is its normal pH?

_____

_____

2. Name five substances that are transported in the blood.

_____

_____

_____

_____

_____

3. In addition to transport, what are five other functions of the blood?

_____

_____

_____

_____

_____

4. What percentage of the blood is plasma? What percentage is formed elements?

_____

5. What is the major component of plasma?

_____

6. What are the three major plasma proteins, and what is the function of each?

_____

_____

_____

7. Identify three types of formed elements, their precursor cells, and the process by which they are formed.

_____

_____

_____

8. Describe the physical characteristics of erythrocytes, and state the normal number.

_____

_____

9. What is the primary function of erythrocytes, and what molecule within the erythrocyte carries out this function?

_____

_____

10. How is the production of erythrocytes regulated, and what three factors are necessary for normal production?

_____

_____

_____

11. What is the normal life span of an erythrocyte, and what happens to its components when it is destroyed?

_____

_____

_____

12. How do the physical characteristics of leukocytes differ from those of erythrocytes?

_____

13. Identify three granulocytes and two agranulocytes, and state the function of each one. Which one is most numerous? Which one is least numerous?

_____

_____

_____

_____

_____

14. What are thrombocytes, and what is their function? How many are normally present in the blood?

_____

_____

15. Define *hemostasis* and describe each of the three processes that contribute to hemostasis.

_____

_____

_____

_____

16. Write three word equations that summarize the steps in coagulation of blood.

_____

_____

_____

17. Name an ion and a vitamin that are necessary for coagulation.

_____

18. As healing progresses, what happens to a blood clot?

_____

19. What agglutinogens and agglutinins are present in each of the five ABO blood types?

_____

_____

_____

20. How do the agglutinogens and agglutinins react in a mismatched transfusion?

_____

21. What ABO blood type is called the universal donor? What type is the universal recipient? Why?

_____

_____

22. What distinguishes Rh+ individuals from Rh− individuals?

_____

_____

23. What happens when an Rh− individual is first exposed to Rh+ blood? What happens when exposed a second time?

_____

_____

_____

_____

24. What is hemolytic disease of the newborn? How does it develop?

_____

_____

_____

_____

25. How is hemolytic disease of the newborn treated? How can it be prevented?

_____

_____

_____

_____

Chapter **13 Cardiovascular System: Blood**

REPRESENTATIVE DISORDERS

Match the disorder of the cardiovascular system on the right with its description on the left.

1. _____ Cancer of blood-forming tissues
2. _____ Increase in number of RBCs
3. _____ Angiitis
4. _____ Deficiency in RBCs or hemoglobin
5. _____ Blood clot
6. _____ Complex of congenital structural heart anomalies
7. _____ Excessive bleeding caused by lack of clotting factors
8. _____ Abnormally decreased amount of circulating plasma
9. _____ Impairment of the conduction system of the heart
10. _____ Degenerative changes in coronary circulation

A. Anemia
B. Coronary artery disease
C. Heart block
D. Hemophilia
E. Hypovolemia
F. Leukemia
G. Polycythemia
H. Tetralogy of Fallot
I. Thrombus
J. Vasculitis

VOCABULARY PRACTICE

Match the definitions on the left with the correct clinical term from the column on the right by placing the corresponding letter in the space before the definition. Not all terms will be used.

1. _____ On the surface of RBCs
2. _____ Stem cell in the bone marrow
3. _____ Blood clot
4. _____ Multiple pinpoint hemorrhages
5. _____ An increase in the number os RBCs
6. _____ Malignant tumor of bone marrow
7. _____ Percentage of RBCs in whole blood
8. _____ Immature RBC
9. _____ Replace clotting factors absent from blood
10. _____ Oral anticoagulant that prevents synthesis of clotting factors

A. Agglutinin
B. Agglutinogen
C. Antihemophilic factors
D. Coumadin
E. Hematocrit
F. Hemocytoblast
G. Heparin
H. Multiple myeloma
I. Polycythemia
J. Purpura
K. Reticulocyte
L. Thrombus

11. Write the meaning of the following abbreviations.

A. _____ CBC
B. _____ PCV
C. _____ Hb
D. _____ HCT or Hct
E. _____ AML

F. _____ EBV
G. _____ PMN
H. _____ WBC
I. _____ CML
J. _____ BMT

12. Spelling is important in scientific and medical applications because only one or two incorrect letters can change the meaning. All of the following words are from this chapter and are spelled incorrectly. Write the correct spelling in the space preceding the misspelled words.

A. _____ dipedesis

B. _____ lukosites

C. _____ hemopoesis

D. _____ agllutination

E. _____ hemolitic

13. Write the meaning of the underlined portion of each word on the line preceding the word.

A. _____ <u>erythro</u>cyte   F. _____ thrombocyto<u>penia</u>

B. _____ mega<u>karyo</u>cyte   G. _____ erythro<u>poietin</u>

C. _____ <u>thrombo</u>cyte   H. _____ baso<u>phil</u>

D. _____ <u>mega</u>karyocyte   I. _____ hemo<u>stasis</u>

E. _____ erythro<u>cyte</u>   J. _____ agg<u>lutino</u>gen

14. For each of the following words, underline the word part that corresponds to the underlined word or phrase in the definition.

A. poikilocytosis   <u>irregularity</u> in the shape of red blood cells

B. leukocyte   <u>white</u> blood cell

C. hemolysis   <u>destruction</u> of red blood cells

D. hemoglobin   <u>protein</u> in red blood cells

E. hemostasis   <u>control</u> or stoppage of bleeding

F. leucopenia   <u>deficiency</u> of leukocytes

G. megakaryocyte   cell with a large lobular <u>nucleus</u> in the bone marrow

H. erythrocyte   <u>red</u> blood cell

I. anticoagulant   substance that inhibits blood <u>clotting</u>

J. hemorrhage   excessive bleeding or <u>flow</u> of blood

Multiple choice: Select the best response.

1. Which one of the following is *not* true about blood? (a) the normal volume of blood is about 5 L, (b) the normal pH of blood is slightly acidic, (c) blood is more viscous than water, (d) blood is classified as a connective tissue.

2. Which one of the following statements about plasma is *not* correct? (a) plasma is about 90% water, (b) fibrinogen is a protein found in plasma, (c) the most abundant plasma proteins are the globulins, (d) some oxygen and carbon dioxide are transported as solutes in the plasma.

3. Normally, the hematocrit of blood is about (a) 45%, (b) 55%, (c) equal to the volume of plasma, (d) 15%.

4. About 60% of the plasma proteins are (a) albumins, (b) fibrinogen, (c) globulins, (d) hemoglobin.

5. The plasma protein that is *not* produced in the liver is (a) fibrinogen, (b) albumin, (c) alpha globulin, (d) gamma globulin.

6. The formed element that is a biconcave disk and has no nucleus is the (a) thrombocyte, (b) basophil, (c) monocyte, (d) erythrocyte.

7. The stem cell for hematopoiesis is the (a) hemocytoblast, (b) megakaryocyte, (c) reticulocyte, (d) proerythroblast.

8. A mineral that is essential for the production of normal hemoglobin is (a) calcium, (b) iron, (c) zinc, (d) magnesium.

9. Two vitamins necessary for the production of normal hemoglobin are (a) vitamin B_{12} and intrinsic factor, (b) folic acid and vitamin D, (c) vitamin B_{12} and folic acid, (d) vitamin D and vitamin K.

10. An inactive form of the hormone erythropoietin, which stimulates the production of erythrocytes, is produced by the (a) liver, (b) kidney, (c) bone marrow, (d) small intestine.

11. Pernicious anemia results from a deficiency of (a) iron, (b) vitamin K, (c) intrinsic factor, (d) heme.

12. When old RBCs are destroyed, the pigment heme portion of hemoglobin is broken down into (a) iron and bilirubin, (b) amino acids, (c) folic acid and iron, (d) vitamin B_{12} and amino acids.

13. Normally, RBCs have a life span of about (a) 2 weeks, (b) 1 month, (c) 1 year, (d) 120 days.

14. The most abundant leukocyte (a) is an agranulocyte, (b) is a lymphocyte, (c) is a neutrophil, (d) has a large nucleus.

15. Phagocytic leukocytes are (a) neutrophils and monocytes, (b) lymphocytes and basophils, (c) basophils and eosinophils, (d) neutrophils and lymphocytes.

16. The leukocyte that produces histamine and heparin is the (a) basophil, (b) eosinophil, (c) neutrophil, (d) lymphocyte.

17. The first event in hemostasis is (b) blood clotting, (b) vascular constriction, (c) formation of a platelet plug, (d) fibrinolysis.

18. The mineral that is essential for normal blood clotting is (a) calcium, (b) iron, (c) potassium, (d) magnesium.

19. The first stage in blood coagulation is the (a) formation of a platelet plug, (b) conversion of prothrombin to thrombin, (c) formation of prothrombin activator, (c) conversion of fibrinogen to fibrin.

20. The basis of blood types is the type of the (a) agglutinogens on the surface of the RBCs, (b) agglutinins on the surface of the RBCs, (c) agglutinogens in the plasma, (d) agglutinins in the plasma.

21. Janie has type O blood. She has (a) type O agglutinogens and no agglutinins, (b) no agglutinogens and type O agglutinins, (c) no agglutinogens and no agglutinins, (d) no agglutinogens and anti-A and anti-B agglutinins.

22. An individual with type A blood may donate blood to (a) type A and type AB individuals; (b) type A and type O individuals; (c) type O and type AB individuals; (d) type B and type AB individuals.

23. An individual with type B blood may receive blood from (a) type A and type AB individuals, (b) type O and type B individuals, (c) type O and type A individuals, (d) type AB and type B individuals.

24. Which of the following statements about Rh blood types is *not* true? (a) about 85% of the population is Rh+; (b) normally, Rh– individuals do not have anti-Rh agglutinins; (c) normally, Rh+ individuals do not have anti-Rh agglutinins; (d) normally, Rh– individuals have Rh– agglutinogens.

25. In blood transfusions, it is always preferable to have and exact match in both the ABO and Rh types. In an emergency, it may be acceptable for a type B+ individual to *receive* (a) type AB+ blood, (b) type AB– blood, (c) type O– blood, (d) type A– blood.

A STEP BEYOND

Go a step beyond the ordinary and learn more about a topic that is related to this chapter but not discussed in detail in the textbook. Select one of the following topics, or one suggested by your instructor, and write a brief paper (250 words minimum), create a poster, or develop a short presentation (approximately 4 to 5 minutes) that focuses on your selection. Suggested topics for this chapter include the following:

1. What is hematopoiesis? Where does it occur? What is the stem cell? What are the intermediate stages between the stem cell and the functional cell types?
2. There are numerous types of anemia, including deficiency anemia, aplastic anemia, hemolytic anemia, sickle cell anemia, and thalassemia. Select any two of these for further study.
3. What is HIV? What is AIDS? How are they related? How are they acquired? How can they be prevented?
4. What is malaria? What is the causative agent? How is it transmitted? What are the effects of malaria?

FUN & GAMES

Word Scramble
Determine the word that fits each definition, and then write the word in the spaces across from the definition, one letter per space. The letters in the boxes form a scrambled word or words. Unscramble the letters to create a word that matches the final definition in each section.

1. Platelet

2. Red blood cells

3. Circulating immature RBCs

4. Liquid portion of blood

Chapter **13** **Cardiovascular System: Blood**

Letters to use for final word: _____

Final definition: Stem cell for formed elements

_____

5. Formation of a blood clot

6. A plasma protein

7. Monocytes in the tissues

8. Predominant plasma protein

Letters to use for final word: _____

Final definition: Blood type antigens

_____

14 Lymphatic System and Immunity

LEARNING EXERCISES
Functions of the Lymphatic System

1. Three functions of the lymphatic system are to:

   A. _____

   B. _____

   C. _____

Components of the Lymphatic System

1. Name the three major components of the lymphatic system.

   A. _____

   B. _____

   C. _____

2. In the spaces on the left, write the answers that match the statements about lymph and lymphatic vessels.

   A. _____   Fluid within the tissue spaces

   B. _____   Source of fluid in tissue spaces

   C. _____   Fluid within lymphatic vessels

   D. _____   Source of fluid within lymphatic vessels

   E. _____   Smallest lymphatic vessels

   F. _____   Largest lymphatic vessels

   G. _____   Drains the upper right quadrant of the body

   H. _____   Collects lymph from ¾ of the body

   I. _____   Structure at beginning of thoracic duct

   J. _____   Returns lymph to right subclavian vein

   K. _____   Returns lymph to left subclavian vein

   L. _____   Prevent backflow of lymph within vessels

M. _____   Actions that move lymph in vessels (3)

_____

_____

3. In the spaces on the left, write the answers that match the statements about the organs of the lymphatic system.

A. _____   Characteristic cells in lymphatic organs

B. _____   Located along lymphatic pathways

C. _____   Located near the mouth, nose, and throat

D. _____   Located posterior to the stomach

E. _____   Located near the heart

F. _____   Filters lymph

G. _____   Filters blood

H. _____   Protect against pathogens that enter via the nose

I. _____   Functions in maturation of T-lymphocytes

J. _____   Reservoir for blood

K. _____   Called *adenoids* when enlarged

L. _____   Carry lymph into a lymph node

M. _____   Hormone from the thymus

N. _____   Consists of red pulp and white pulp

Resistance to Disease

1. In the spaces on the left, write the words that are defined on the right.

A. _____   Disease-producing organisms

B. _____   Ability to counteract harmful agents

C. _____   Lack of resistance

D. _____   Mechanisms against all harmful agents

E. _____   Mechanisms against selected harmful agents

F. _____   Specific resistance

2. Systemic inflammation is a medical crisis. List three characteristics of systemic inflammation.

A. _____

B. _____

C. _____

3. Match each of the following processes, agents, and components with the nonspecific defense mechanism of which it is a part.

A. _____ Unbroken skin and mucous membranes

B. _____ Activates phagocytosis and inflammation

C. _____ Blocks replication of viruses

D. _____ Cilia action in the respiratory tract

E. _____ Interferon

F. _____ Accompanied by swelling, heat, and redness

G. _____ Ingestion and destruction of solid particles by certain cells

H. _____ Action of complement

I. _____ Macrophages and neutrophils

J. _____ Aimed at localizing damage and destroying its source

1. barrier to entry

2. protective chemical action

3. phagocytosis

4. inflammatory reaction

4. In the spaces on the left, write the answers that match the statements about specific defense mechanisms.

A. _____   Characteristics of immunity (2)

_____

B. _____   Primary cell types involved in immunity (2)

_____

C. _____   Molecules that trigger immune responses

D. _____   Lymphocytes that mature in the thymus

E. _____   30% of circulating lymphocytes

F. _____   Responsible for cell-mediated immunity

G. _____   Mature someplace other than in the thymus

H. _____   Responsible for humoral immunity

I. _____   70% of circulating lymphocytes

J. _____   Produce antibodies

K. _____   Another term for antibodies

Chapter 14 Lymphatic System and Immunity

L. _____   Initial action against antigens

M. _____   Subgroups of T cells (4)

_____

_____

_____

N. _____   Clones of B cells (2)

_____

5. Write IgG, IgA, IgM, IgD, or IgE on the line preceding each phrase to identify the class of antibodies it describes.

A. _____   Most numerous antibody

B. _____   Responsible for allergic reactions

C. _____   Found in breast milk, saliva, mucus, and tears

D. _____   Responsible for ABO transfusion reactions

E. _____   Major antibody in immune responses

F. _____   Binds to mast cells and causes release of histamine

G. _____   Crosses placenta to provide immunity for newborn

H. _____   Causes agglutination of antigens

Match each of the following descriptions with the type of immunity it characterizes.

A. active natural   B. active artificial   C. passive natural   D. passive artificial

6. _____   Antiserum is injected into an individual.

7. _____   A person contracts a disease, recovers, and is immune to that disease.

8. _____   Antibodies are transferred from one person to another through natural processes.

9. _____   Antigens deliberately introduced into a person to stimulate immunity

10. _____   Memory cells produced after contracting a disease such as chickenpox

11. _____   Antibodies injected into an individual after a poisonous snakebite

12. _____   IgA antibodies in mother's milk may provide some immunity for infants.

13. _____   Mumps, diphtheria, whooping cough, and tetanus vaccines

REVIEW QUESTIONS

1. What are the three primary functions of the lymphatic system?

   _____

2. What three basic components make up the lymphatic system?

   _____

   _____

3. What is lymph?

   _____

   _____

4. What part of the body is drained by the thoracic duct? What part is drained by the right lymphatic duct?

   _____

   _____

   _____

5. There is no pump to move fluid through the lymphatic vessels. What provides the pressure gradients that are necessary to move the lymph?

   _____

   _____

6. For what purpose and by what pathway does lymph flow through lymph nodes?

   _____

   _____

   _____

7. What is the purpose of tonsils, and where are they located?

   _____

   _____

   _____

8. What structural feature of the spleen characterizes it as a lymphatic organ? List two functions of the spleen.

   _____

   _____

   _____

9. When is the thymus most active, and what is its function?

_____

_____

_____

10. Use the term *pathogen* in a definition of resistance.

_____

11. What is meant when a defense mechanism is said to be nonspecific? Give an example.

_____

_____

12. Give an example of a mechanical barrier that inhibits the entry of pathogens.

_____

13. What is the particular significance of interferon in body defense?

_____

14. What is the role of neutrophils and macrophages in body defense?

_____

15. What are the four characteristics of localized inflammation? What are three additional characteristics of systemic inflammation?

_____

_____

_____

_____

_____

_____

16. In addition to their specificity, what is another feature of specific defense mechanisms?

_____

17. What is an antigen?

_____

18. What percentage of the circulating lymphocytes are normally T cells? Where do they differentiate into T cells?

_____

_____

19. What four clones of cells are produced in cell-mediated immunity?

_____

_____

_____

_____

20. What is the function of plasma cells, and with what specific type of immunity are they associated?

_____

_____

21. In antibody-mediated immunity, which is more rapid—the primary response or the secondary response?

_____

_____

22. What is the meaning of the abbreviation *Ig*?

_____

23. Which type of immunoglobulin is most numerous in blood plasma?

_____

24. What is the source of antibodies in passive immunity?

_____

25. An individual receives a vaccination that contains a specially prepared antigen. What type of immunity is acquired through this procedure?

_____

FUNCTIONAL RELATIONSHIPS

It is important to remember that no system in the body works alone. It takes the interaction of all systems to maintain homeostasis. The following exercises reinforce the concept that all systems work together to maintain the health and well-being of other systems and the individual.

Match the system on the right with what it provides for the lymphatic system on the left. Use the functional relationships page in your concepts textbook as a resource.

1. _____ Provides mechanical barrier to pathogens

2. _____ Protects thymus and spleen

3. _____ Moves lymph within vessels

4. _____ Innervates lymphoid organs

5. _____ Products suppress immune response

6. _____ Transports oxygen and nutrients to lymphoid organs

7. _____ Provides oxygen for lymphoid organs

8. _____ Absorbs nutrients needed by lymphoid tissue

9. _____ Helps maintain fluid, electrolyte, and pH balance for effective immune function

10. _____ Acidic secretions provide a barrier against infections

A. Cardiovascular

B. Digestive

C. Endocrine

D. Integumentary

E. Muscular

F. Nervous

G. Reproductive

H. Respiratory

I. Skeletal

J. Urinary

11. For each of the following systems, write what the lymphatic system provides for it.

A. Cardiovascular _____

B. Skeletal _____

C. Reproductive _____

D. Endocrine _____

E. Respiratory _____

F. Muscular _____

G. Nervous _____

H. Digestive _____

I. Urinary _____

J. Integumentary _____

REPRESENTATIVE DISORDERS

Match the disorder of the lymphatic system on the right with its description of the left.

1. _____ Inflammation and enlargement of tonsils

2. _____ Characterized by a systemic vasodilation with a dramatic decrease in blood pressure

3. _____ Inhibition of the formation of antibodies

4. _____ Most common form is poison ivy

5. _____ Disease of lymph nodes

6. _____ Autoimmune disease

7. _____ Late stage of HIV infection

8. _____ Virus that destroys helper T cells

9. _____ Enlargement of the spleen

10. _____ Malignant tumor of lymph nodes

A. AIDS

B. Anaphylaxis

C. Contact dermatitis

D. HIV

E. Immunosuppression

F. Lymphadenopathy

G. Lymphoma

H. Rheumatoid arthritis

I. Splenomegaly

J. Tonsillitis

VOCABULARY PRACTICE

Match the definitions on the left with the correct clinical term from the column on the right by placing the corresponding letter in the space before the definition. Not all terms will be used.

1. _____ A substance that triggers an immune response

2. _____ Immunity produced when antibodies are passes through breast milk from mother to infant

3. _____ Used to reduce rejection of kidney and liver transplants

4. _____ Specialist in the diagnosis and treatment of malignant disorders

5. _____ Malignant tumor of lymph nodes/lymph tissue

6. _____ Ability to counteract the effects of pathogens

7. _____ Preparations that contain antibodies

8. _____ An exaggerated or unusual hypersensitivity reaction to a foreign protein

9. _____ Spread of a tumor to a secondary site

10. _____ Enlargement of the spleen

A. Anaphylaxis

B. Antibody

C. Antigen

D. Antisera

E. Artificial

F. Immunosuppressants

G. Lymphoma

H. Metastasis

I. Oncologist

J. Passive

K. Resistance

L. Splenomegaly

M. Susceptibility

N. Toxoids

11. Write the meaning of the following abbreviations.

A. _____ AIDS

B. _____ CMV

C. _____ KS

D. _____ HIV

E. _____ IDC

F. _____ DCIS

G. _____ HSV

H. _____ Ig

I. _____ ELISA

J. _____ NHL

12. Spelling is important in scientific and medical applications because only one or two incorrect letters can change the meaning. All of the following words are from this chapter, but only two are spelled incorrectly. Place a check (✓) in the space preceding the words that are spelled correctly. Write the correct spelling in the space preceding the misspelled words.

A. _____ immunoglobulins

B. _____ eferent

C. _____ vaccination

D. _____ pyrogens

E. _____ thorasic

13. Write the meaning of the underlined portion of each word on the line preceding the word.

A. _____ <u>tox</u>oid

B. _____ <u>immun</u>ology

C. _____ hemo<u>lytic</u>

D. _____ <u>onc</u>ology

E. _____ <u>lymph</u>angiography

14. Separate the following words into their component parts, give the definition of each part, and then put the parts together to write a definition for the entire word.

A. lymphadenopathy

_____

B. splenorrhagia

_____

15. Mary Lynn Fatic was diagnosed with breast cancer and had a portion of the breast tissue removed. During the procedure, the surgeon also excised the axillary lymph nodes. After the surgery, she developed swelling in her arm.

A. Why were the lymph nodes removed?

_____

_____

B. What caused the swelling in the arm?

_____

_____

C. What is the medical term for the swelling she experienced?

_____

TESTING COMPREHENSION

Multiple choice: Select the best response.

1. Which of the following is *not* a function of the lymphatic system? (a) return carbon dioxide from the tissues to the blood, (b) defense against invading microorganisms, (c) absorption of fats and fat-soluble vitamins, (d) return excess interstitial fluid to the blood.

2. The lymphatic vessel that drains lymph from the entire body except the upper right quadrant is the (a) right lymphatic duct, (b) lacteal, (c) cisterna chyli, (d) thoracic duct.

3. The beginning of the thoracic duct is the (a) lacteal, (b) cisterna chyli, (c) villus, (d) lymph capillary.

4. An obstruction to lymph flow may cause an increase in (a) plasma proteins, (b) interstitial fluid or edema, (c) hematocrit, (d) plasma volume.

5. The largest lymphatic vessel is the (a) thoracic duct, (b) right lymphatic duct, (c) lymphatic trunk, (d) lumbar trunk.

6. The primary function of lymph nodes is to (a) filter and cleanse the blood, (b) produce lymphocytes, (c) filter and cleanse the lymph, (d) act as a reservoir for lymph.

7. Lymph nodes are not found in the (a) axilla, (b) inguinal area, (c) neck, (d) central nervous system.

8. Lymph nodes typically have (a) one efferent vessel and one afferent vessel, (b) one efferent vessel and multiple afferent vessels, (c) multiple efferent vessels and one afferent vessel, (d) multiple efferent vessels and multiple afferent vessels.

9. Clusters of lymphatic tissue under the mucous membranes of the nose, mouth, and throat are the (a) tonsils, (b) thymus, (c) lymph nodes, (d) cisterna chyli.

10. Nate had an adenoidectomy when he was a child. What was surgically excised? (a) lingual tonsils, (b) thymus, (c) pharyngeal tonsils, (d) palatine tonsils.

11. The largest lymphatic organ in the body is (a) a lymph node, (b) a tonsil, (c) the thymus, (d) the spleen.

12. Which of the following is *not* a function of the spleen? (a) filter and cleanse blood, (b) produce lymphocytes, (c) act as a reservoir for blood, (d) filter and cleanse lymph.

13. First-line barriers in nonspecific defense against disease include (a) complement and interferon, (b) unbroken skin and lysozymes, (c) phagocytosis and inflammation, (d) unbroken skin and inflammation.

14. Second-line barriers in nonspecific defense against disease include (a) phagocytosis and inflammation, (b) lysozymes and interferon, (c) complement and fluid flow, (d) mucous membranes and phagocytosis.

15. The phagocytes in lymphoid tissue are (a) neutrophils and lymphocytes, (b) lymphocytes and macrophages, (c) neutrophils and macrophages, (d) lymphocytes and eosinophils.

16. The effects of localized inflammation include (a) a dangerous decrease in blood pressure, (b) stimulation of the bone marrow, (c) an increase in capillary permeability, (d) an increase in metabolic rate.

17. Which of the following does *not* pertain to systemic inflammation? (a) it is aimed at localized tissue damage and destroying its source, (b) it includes leukocytosis, (c) pyrogens cause a fever, (d) capillary permeability may be so generalized there is a dangerous decrease in blood pressure.

18. A molecule that triggers and immune response is (a) an antibody, (b) an antigen, (c) a pyrogen, (d) a plasma cell.

19. Clones of B cells include (a) killer cells, (b) helper cells, (c) plasma cells, (d) suppressor cells.

20. The lymphocytes responsible for cell-mediated immunity become differentiated in the (a) spleen, (b) liver, (c) lymph nodes, (d) thymus.

21. Antibodies are produced by (a) T cells, (b) memory cells, (c) helper cells, (d) plasma cells.

22. The major immunoglobulin in primary and secondary responses is (a) IgG, (b) IgA, (c) IgE, (d) IgD.

23. The rapid secondary response is due to (a) plasma cells, (b) killer cells, (c) memory cells, (d) helper cells.

24. Vaccinations are used to develop (a) active natural immunity, (b) active artificial immunity, (c) passive natural immunity, (d) passive acquired immunity.

25. An antiserum is used to provide (a) active natural immunity, (b) active artificial immunity, (c) passive natural immunity, (d) passive artificial immunity.

A STEP BEYOND

Go a step beyond the ordinary and learn more about a topic that is related to this chapter but not discussed in detail in the textbook. Select one of the following topics, or one suggested by your instructor, and write a brief paper (250 words minimum), create a poster, or develop a short presentation (approximately 4 to 5 minutes) that focuses on your selection. Suggested topics for this chapter:

1. What is interferon? What is its use? How can it be produced in usable quantity? What is the focus of current research regarding interferon?
2. What are vaccinations? How are they used? What is their value? What is the nature of the vaccine? Are there any arguments against vaccinations?
3. What is anaphylaxis? Who is susceptible? Why is anaphylaxis a medical crisis? What can be done to prevent its occurrence? How is it treated?
4. Do you have some type of allergy? Learn about your allergy. What is the allergen? What are its physiologic effects? What are the mechanisms that result in these effects?

FUN & GAMES

Word Scramble

Determine the word that fits each definition, and then write the word in the spaces across from the definition, one letter per space. The letters in the boxes form a scrambled word or words. Unscramble the letters to create a word that matches the final definition in each section.

1. An antigen that causes a specific hypersensitivity

2. Spread of a malignant tumor to a secondary site

3. Small phagocytic cells

4. First line of nonspecific defense

☐☐☐☐☐☐

5. Specific resistance

☐☐☐☐☐☐

6. Enlarged pharyngeal tonsils

☐☐☐☐☐☐

Letters to use for final word: _____

Final definition: Antibodies

_____

7. Immunity that is the opposite of active

☐☐☐☐☐☐

8. A specialist in the diagnosis and treatment of malignant disorders

☐☐☐☐☐☐☐☐☐

9. Immunity that is not natural

☐☐☐☐☐☐☐

10. An agent that causes fever

☐☐☐☐☐☐

Letters to use for final word: _____

Final definition: Infection to stimulate active artificial immunity

_____

LEARNING EXERCISES

Functions and Overview of Respiration

1. In the spaces on the left, write the terms that match the phrases about the sequence of events in respiration.

A. _____ Exchange of air between atmosphere and lungs

B. _____ Exchange of gases between lungs and blood

C. _____ Function of blood in respiration

D. _____ Exchange of gases between blood and tissues

E. _____ Utilization of oxygen in the cells

Ventilation

1. Use the letter *U* to designate the regions of the upper respiratory tract and the letter *L* to designate the regions of the lower respiratory tract.

A. _____ Bronchi   D. _____ Pharynx

B. _____ Nose   E. _____ Lungs

C. _____ Larynx   F. _____ Trachea

2. In the spaces on the left, write the answers that match the phrases about the respiratory tract.

A. _____   Functions of the nasal cavity (3)

_____

_____

B. _____   Region of pharynx posterior to the nasal cavity

C. _____   Location of the pharyngeal tonsils

D. _____   Pharynx from the uvula to the hyoid bone

E. _____   Lowest region of the pharynx

F. _____   Cartilage that forms the Adam's apple

G. _____   Most inferior cartilage of the larynx

H. _____   Prevents food from entering the larynx

I. _____ Opening between the true vocal cords

J. _____ Passage commonly called the windpipe

K. _____ Ridge of cartilage at bifurcation of the trachea

L. _____ Tissue that forms lining of the trachea

M. _____ Tissue that forms the alveoli

3. Arrange the following air passages in the correct sequence from largest to smallest by placing the numbers 1 to 7 in the spaces before the names. Use number 1 for the largest and number 7 for the smallest.

A. _____ Alveolar ducts   E. _____ Lobar bronchi

B. _____ Respiratory bronchioles F. _____ Terminal bronchioles

C. _____ Alveoli   G. _____ Primary bronchi

D. _____ Segmental bronchi

4. Place an R in the space preceding the phrase if it refers to the right lung. Place an L in the space if it refers to the left lung. If the phrase applies to both lungs, place a B in the space.

A. _____ Cardiac notch   E. _____ Rests on the diaphragm

B. _____ Two lobes   F. _____ Has two fissures

C. _____ Shorter and wider   G. _____ Enclosed by the pleura

D. _____ Divided into lobules   H. _____ Anchored at the root or hilum

5. In the spaces on the left, write the answers that match the phrases about pulmonary ventilation.

A. _____ Name of pressure between layers of pleurae

B. _____ Name of pressure outside the body

C. _____ Name of pressure within the alveoli

D. _____ Pressure that is normally less than the two others

E. _____ Primary muscle involved in quiet breathing

F. _____ Muscles used in forced expiration

G. _____ Reduces surface tension within the alveoli

H. _____ Instrument to measure respiratory volumes

I. _____ Highest pressure during expiration

J. _____ Highest pressure during inspiration

6. Write *I* in the space if the event occurs during inspiration, and write *E* if it occurs during expiration.

A. _____ Diaphragm contracts

B. _____ Intrapulmonary pressure exceeds atmospheric pressure

C. _____ External intercostal muscles may contract

D. _____ Atmospheric pressure is greater than intrapulmonary pressure

E. _____ Lung volume increases

F. _____ Diaphragm relaxes

G. _____ Internal intercostal muscles may contract

H. _____ Air flows into the lungs

I. _____ Elastic recoil decreases the size of the alveoli

7. Match the lung volumes and capacities with their definitions.

TV = tidal volume   VC = vital capacity
IRV = inspiratory reserve volume   IC = inspiratory capacity
ERV = expiratory reserve volume   FRC = functional residual capacity
RV = residual volume   TLC = total lung capacity

A. _____ Maximum amount of air that can be inhaled

B. _____ Amount of air inhaled and exhaled in a quiet breathing cycle

C. _____ Amount of air in lungs after quiet expiration

D. _____ Equals TV + IRV + ERV

E. _____ Maximum amount of air that can be inhaled after a tidal inspiration

F. _____ Amount of air in lungs after maximum inspiration

G. _____ Maximum amount of air that can be forcefully exhaled after tidal expiration

H. _____ Equals RV + ERV

I. _____ Amount of air in lungs after maximum expiration

J. _____ Equals RV + ERV + TV + IRV

8. Complete the following table by writing in the correct values in the blank spaces.

TLC	VC	TV	ERV	IRV	RV
		500 mL	1000 mL	3000 mL	1200 mL
6000 mL	5000 mL		900 mL	3500 mL	
	4700 mL	600 mL	800 mL		1100 mL
5900 mL	4600 mL	400 mL		3000 mL	

9. If the individual type on the left tends to have greater lung volume than the type on the right, write > (greater than) on the blank in the center. If the left type tends to have less lung volume than the type on the right, write < (less than).

A. Young adults   _____   Senior citizens

B. Females   _____   Males

C. Short people   _____   Tall people

D. Normal weight people   _____   Obese people

E. Healthy people   _____   People with muscular disease

F. People in good physical condition   _____   People in poor physical condition

Basic Gas Laws and Respiration

1. Atmospheric air is a mixture of oxygen, nitrogen, and carbon dioxide. According to Dalton's law of partial pressures, if the atmospheric pressure is 750 mm Hg and the oxygen content is 21%, what is the pressure due to oxygen?

_____

2. According to Henry's law, what two factors determine how much of each gas in a mixture will dissolve in a liquid?

_____

3. Complete the following statements that define external and internal respiration.

External respiration is the exchange of gases between the _____ and the

_____.

Internal respiration is the exchange of gases between the _____ and the

_____.

4. List, in sequence, the six layers of the respiratory membrane through which oxygen must pass to diffuse from the alveolus into the blood capillary.

A.

B.

C.

D.

E.

F.

5. Indicate whether each of the following will increase or decrease the rate of gaseous exchange across the respiratory membrane. Use *I* for increase and *D* for decrease.

A. _____ Decreasing the surface area of the respiratory membrane

B. _____ Fluid accumulation in the alveoli resulting from pulmonary edema

C. _____ Increasing tidal volume

D. _____ Decreasing breathing rate

Transport of Gases

1. List two ways in which oxygen is transported in the blood.

_____

_____

2. List three ways in which carbon dioxide is transported in the blood.

_____

_____

_____

3. In the spaces on the left, write the answers that match the phrases about oxygen and carbon dioxide transport.

A. _____ Compound in which most oxygen is transported

B. _____ Method of most carbon dioxide transport

C. _____ Combination of carbon dioxide and hemoglobin

D. _____ Combination of water and carbon dioxide

E. _____ Enzyme that speeds up the reaction between water and carbon dioxide

4. Place a check (✓) in front of the factors in the tissues that favor unloading of oxygen.

A. _____ Increased partial pressure of oxygen

B. _____ Increased partial pressure of carbon dioxide

C. _____ Increased hydrogen ion concentration

D. _____ Increased temperature

E. _____ Increased pH

F. _____ Increased cellular metabolism

5. Place an E before the phrases that refer to external respiration, and place an I before the phrases that refer to internal respiration.

   A. _____ Oxygen diffuses into the blood

   B. _____ Oxygen diffuses out of the blood

   C. _____ Carbon dioxide diffuses into the blood

   D. _____ Carbon dioxide diffuses out of the blood

   E. _____ Occurs in the alveolus

   F. _____ Occurs in the body tissues

   G. _____ Bicarbonate ion is formed

   H. _____ Bicarbonate ions release carbon dioxide

   I. _____ Oxyhemoglobin is formed

   J. _____ Oxyhemoglobin dissociates and releases oxygen

Regulation of Respiration

1. The respiratory center includes neurons in the _____ and

   _____.

2. The inspiratory areas of the respiratory center send impulses along the _____

   nerve to the diaphragm and along the _____ nerves to the external intercostal
   muscles.

3. Place a *T* before each true statement and an *F* before each false statement about factors that influence the rate and depth of breathing.

   A. _____ Chemoreceptors in the medulla oblongata are sensitive to changes in oxygen levels.

   B. _____ Increases in blood CO_2 levels increase the rate and depth of breathing.

   C. _____ Increases in hydrogen ion concentrations increase the rate and depth of breathing.

   D. _____ Chemoreceptors in the medulla oblongata are sensitive to changes in carbon dioxide and hydrogen ion concentrations.

   E. _____ A decrease in oxygen levels is usually a strong stimulus for breathing.

   F. _____ Decreased oxygen levels usually make the respiratory center more sensitive to carbon dioxide changes.

   G. _____ Peripheral chemoreceptors are located in the aortic and carotid bodies.

   H. _____ The Hering-Breuer reflex prevents overinflation of the lungs.

   I. _____ The Hering-Breuer reflex is a response to stretch receptors in the lungs.

   J. _____ Higher brain centers may permanently override the respiratory center.

K. _____ Anxiety decreases the rate and depth of breathing.

L. _____ Chronic pain stimulates breathing, but sudden pain may cause a momentary cessation of breathing.

M. _____ Decreasing body temperature increases the breathing rate.

N. _____ The primary stimulus for breathing is decreased carbon dioxide levels in the respiratory center.

LABELING & COLORING EXERCISES

1. Figure 15-1 illustrates the conducting passages of the respiratory tract. Color the upper respiratory tract green and the lower respiratory tract yellow. Identify structures as indicated.

A. _____

B. _____

C. _____

D. _____

E. _____

F. _____

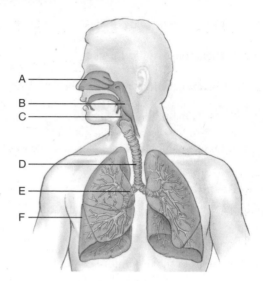

Figure 15-1   Respiratory tract.

2. Figure 15-2 illustrates some of the features of the upper respiratory tract. Color the two sinuses yellow and the tonsils red. Identify structures as indicated.

A. _____

B. _____

C. _____

D. _____

E. _____

F. _____

G. _____

H. _____

I. _____

J. _____

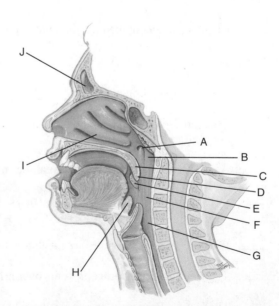

Figure 15-2   Upper respiratory tract.

212

3. Figure 15-3 represents a graph of respiratory volumes and capacities as recorded by a spirometer. Color the portion that represents tidal volume red. Identify the other volumes and capacities as indicated.

A. _____

B. _____

C. _____

D. _____

E. _____

F. _____

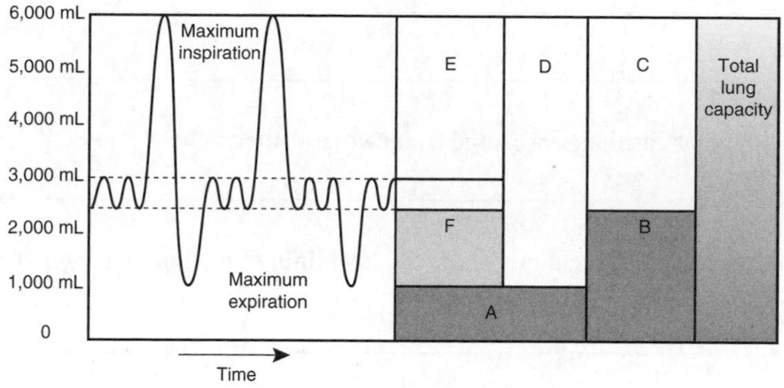

Figure 15-3   Respiratory volumes and capacities.

REVIEW QUESTIONS

1. List the five activities of the total respiratory process.

_____

_____

2. What structures are in the upper respiratory tract? Which ones are in the lower respiratory tract?

_____

_____

3. What are the external nares, internal nares, hard palate, soft palate, uvula, and nasal conchae?

_____

_____

_____

_____

_____

_____

4. What are the functions of the nasal cavity?

_____

_____

5. In what specific regions of the pharynx are the pharyngeal, palatine, and lingual tonsils located?

_____

_____

6. What are the three largest cartilages in the larynx?

_____

_____

_____

7. What type of cartilage forms the framework of the trachea?

_____

8. What two structural features of the tracheal lining function to prevent dirt and other particles from entering the lower respiratory tract?

_____

_____

9. Trace the branching of the bronchial tree from the trachea to the alveoli in the lungs.

_____

_____

_____

10. What structural feature of the alveoli permits the rapid diffusion of gases?

_____

11. How many lobes are in the right lung? Left lung?

_____

_____

12. What is between the parietal pleura and the visceral pleura?

_____

_____

13. During inspiration, which one of the three pressures involved in pulmonary ventilation is the greatest?

_____

14. Why is inspiration considered an active process and expiration a passive process?

_____

_____

15. What substance reduces surface tension within the alveoli?

_____

16. Identify four respiratory volumes and four respiratory capacities on a spirogram.

_____

_____

_____

_____

17. How do age, sex, body build, and physical conditioning affect lung volumes and capacities?

_____

_____

_____

_____

18. What two properties of gases (gas laws) have an effect on the diffusion of a gas?

_____

_____

19. A molecule of oxygen diffuses from the alveolus to capillary blood during external respiration. Name, in sequence, the six layers it must pass through.

_____

_____

_____

_____

_____

_____

20. If the thickness of the respiratory membrane increases and other factors remain constant, how is the rate of external respiration affected?

_____

_____

21. Where does internal respiration take place?

_____

_____

22. How does an increase in carbon dioxide concentration affect the ability of oxygen to combine with hemoglobin?

_____

_____

23. Which normally provides more stimulus for breathing—a decrease in oxygen or an increase in carbon dioxide?

_____

24. How is most of the carbon dioxide transported by the blood?

_____

25. Where is the respiratory center located in the brain?

_____

26. What nerve sends inspiratory impulses to the diaphragm? To the external intercostal muscles?

_____

_____

_____

FUNCTIONAL RELATIONSHIPS

It is important to remember that no system in the body works alone. It takes the interaction of all systems to maintain homeostasis. The following exercises reinforce the concept that all systems work together to maintain the health and wellbeing of other systems and the individual.

Match the system on the right with what it provides for the respiratory system on the left. Use the functional relationships page in your concepts textbook as a resource.

1. _____   Helps maintain body temperature

2. _____   Encloses the lungs for protection

3. _____   Creates pressure changes necessary for ventilation

4. _____   Controls rate and depth of breathing

5. _____   Epinephrine stimulates bronchodilation

6. _____   Transports oxygen and carbon dioxide

7. _____   IgA protects respiratory mucosa

8. _____   Absorbs nutrients for cell maintenance

9. _____   Eliminates waste products generated by respiratory system

10. _____   Sexual arousal stimulates changes in rate and depth of breathing

A. Cardiovascular
B. Digestive
C. Endocrine
D. Integumentary
E. Lymphatic
F. Muscular
G. Nervous
H. Reproductive
I. Skeletal
J. Urinary

2. For each of the following systems, write what the respiratory system provides for it.

A. Cardiovascular   _____

_____

B. Skeletal   _____

C. Reproductive _____

_____

D. Endocrine _____

_____

E. Lymphatic _____

_____

F. Muscular _____

G. Nervous _____

_____

H. Digestive _____

_____

I. Urinary _____

J. Integumentary _____

REPRESENTATIVE DISORDERS

Match the disorder of the respiratory system on the right with its description of the left.

1. _____ Hereditary disorder characterized by the accumulation of excessively thick and adhesive mucus

2. _____ Excessive pressure in the pulmonary arteries

3. _____ Accumulation of fluid in the space between the visceral and parietal layers of pleura

4. _____ Recurrent attacks of difficult breathing because of spasmodic constriction of the bronchi

5. _____ Terminal bronchioles become plugged with mucus, lung tissue loses elasticity, and expiration becomes difficult

6. _____ Lung pathology that occurs after long-term inhalation of pollutants

7. _____ Accumulation of air in the pleural space

8. _____ Abnormality in surfactant that causes alveoli to collapse; often occurs in infants

9. _____ Inflammation of one or more bronchi

10. _____ Infectious, inflammatory disease of the lungs

A. Asthma

B. Bronchitis

C. Cystic fibrosis

D. Emphysema

E. Pleural effusion

F. Pneumoconiosis

G. Pneumothorax

H. Pulmonary hypertension

I. Respiratory distress syndrome

J. Tuberculosis

Match the definitions on the left with the correct clinical term from the column on the right by placing the corresponding letter in the space before the definition. Not all terms will be used.

1. _____ Movement of air into and out of the lungs

2. _____ Inflammation of the diaphragm

3. _____ Accumulation of air in the pleural space

4. _____ Whooping cough

5. _____ Suppress the cough reflex in the medulla oblongata

6. _____ Exchange of gases between the lungs and blood

7. _____ Spitting of blood from bleeding in the respiratory tract

8. _____ Common cold

9. _____ Swelling and fluid in the alveoli and bronchioles

10. _____ Break down mucus and promote coughing

A. Antitussives

B. Atelectasis

C. Coryza

D. External respiration

E. Hemoptysis

F. Internal respiration

G. Mucolytics

H. Pertussis

I. Phrenitis

J. Pneumothorax

K. Pulmonary edema

L. Ventilation

11. Write the meaning of the following abbreviations.

A. _____ VC

B. _____ COPD

C. _____ IPPB

D. _____ RDS

E. _____ TB

F. _____ DPT

G. _____ CPAP

H. _____ SIDS

I. _____ CF

J. _____ OSA

12. Spelling is important in scientific and medical applications because only one or two incorrect letters can change the meaning. Circle the correctly spelled word for each of the following pairs.

A. intraalveolar   intralveolar

B. diaphram   diaphragm

C. larynx   larnyx

D. pleura   plura

E. emphysemia   emphysema

13. Write the meaning of the underlined portion of each word on the line preceding the word.

    A. _____ pneumo<u>con</u>iosis

    B. _____ hyper<u>capn</u>ia

    C. _____ <u>rhino</u>plasty

    D. _____ atel<u>ectasis</u>

    E. _____ dys<u>pnea</u>

    F. _____ hemo<u>ptysis</u>

    G. _____ dys<u>phonia</u>

    H. _____ rhino<u>rrhea</u>

    I. _____ bronchi<u>ole</u>

    J. _____ anthra<u>cosis</u>

14. For each of the following words, underline the word part that corresponds to the underlined word or phrase in the definition.

    A. atelectasis   <u>incomplete</u> dilation of a lung, collapsed lung

    B. dyspnea   labored or <u>difficult</u> breathing

    C. respiration   <u>act of</u> breathing

    D. rhinoplasty   plastic surgery of the <u>nose</u>

    E. bronchiectasis   chronic <u>dilation</u> of the bronchi

    F. pneumomycosis   any fungal disease of the <u>lung</u>

    G. eupnea   normal of <u>good</u> breathing

    H. phonation   <u>voice</u> production

    I. cricoid   laryngeal cartilage that resembles a <u>ring</u>

    J. rhinorrhea   free <u>discharge</u> of a thin nasal mucus

15. Russ P. Tory worked in an environment with high levels of dust pollution. After several years, he developed shortness of breath, chronic cough, and expectoration of mucus containing particles of dust. His condition forced him to quit his job. What is the medical word for this group of lung diseases?

_____

Multiple choice: Select the best response.

1. The act of breathing is called (a) external respiration, (b) ventilation, (c) internal respiration, (d) phonation.

2. The nostrils are also called the (a) internal nares, (b) fauces, (c) external nares, (d) conchae.

3. The pathway of inhaled air is (a) nasal cavity, trachea, larynx, bronchi, pharynx, alveoli; (b) nasal cavity, pharynx, larynx, trachea, bronchi, alveoli; (c) nasal cavity, larynx, pharynx, trachea, bronchi, alveoli; (d) nasal cavity, pharynx, trachea, bronchi, larynx, alveoli.

4. The following pairs of terms indicate a region of the pharynx and a structure or opening associated with that region. Which pair is *not* matched correctly? (a) nasopharynx/openings for auditory tubes, (b) oropharynx/fauces, (c) oropharynx/palatine tonsils, (d) laryngopharynx/pharyngeal tonsils.

5. The largest cartilage of the larynx is the (a) thyroid cartilage, (b) cricoid cartilage, (c) arytenoid cartilage, (d) corniculate cartilage.

6. Which of the following is *not* correct about the trachea? (a) it begins just inferior to the cricoid cartilage; (b) it consists of 15 to 20 complete rings of hyaline cartilage; (c) the lining is ciliated pseudostratified columnar epithelium; (d) it bifurcates at a region called the *carina*.

7. Which of the following is correct about the lungs and pleura? (a) the left lung has three lobes and is longer than the right lung; (b) the pleural cavity is between the visceral pleura and the alveoli; (c) the heart makes an indentation called the cardiac notch in the right lung; (d) the lungs are divided into bronchopulmonary segments, each with its own segmental bronchus.

8. The pressure within the pleural cavity is normally (a) greater than the atmospheric pressure but less than the pressure in the alveoli, (b) less than both atmospheric pressure and intrapulmonary pressure, (c) less than atmospheric pressure but greater than intraalveolar pressure, (d) equal to intrapulmonary pressure.

9. If air or fluid accumulates in the pleural cavity so that the pressure increases above intra-alveolar pressure, the (a) lungs collapse, (b) surfactant is destroyed, (c) fluid or air enters the lungs, (d) person inhales.

10. During expiration, the (a) diaphragm contracts, (b) external intercostals muscles contract, (c) internal intercostals muscles relax, (d) the diaphragm relaxes.

11. Given that atmospheric pressure is 760 mm Hg, intra-alveolar pressure is 763 mm Hg and intrapleural pressure is 756 mm Hg, which of the following is indicated? (a) inspiration phase of ventilation, (b) expiration phase of ventilation, (c) period after expiration but before next inspiration, (d) the lungs are collapsed.

12. Jose was tested with a spirometer. His tidal volume = 450 mL, inspiratory reserve volume = 2800 mL, expiratory reserve volume = 1050 mL, and residual volume = 1200 mL. What was Jose's vital capacity? (a) 1500 mL, (b) 3250 mL, (c) 5500 mL, (d) 4300 mL.

13. Inspiratory capacity equals (a) TV + IRV, (b) IRV + ERV, (c) IRV + FRC, (d) TV + EVR.

14. If you leave an open can of carbonated beverage on the table for an extended time, it loses its carbon dioxide or goes "flat." This is based on (a) Boyle's law, (b) Dalton's law, (c) Henry's law, (d) Hering-Breuer's law.

15. Assume that you are at an elevation where the atmospheric pressure is 700 mm Hg, the air is 79% nitrogen, and the remainder is oxygen. What is the O_2 partial pressure? (a) 21%, (b) 553 mm Hg, (c) 621 mm Hg, (d) 147 mm Hg.

16. Which of the following is *not* true about external respiration? (a) carbon dioxide enters the blood and oxygen enters the alveoli, (b) gases diffuse across the respiratory membrane in the lungs, (c) an accumulation of fluid in the alveoli decreases the diffusion rate, (d) surface area affects the diffusion rate.

17. Which of the following is true about internal respiration? (a) gases diffuse across the respiratory membrane in the lungs, (b) internal respiration occurs in the lungs and external respiration occurs when air enters the nasal cavity, (c) oxygen diffuses from the capillaries into the tissue cells, (d) carbon dioxide diffuses from the blood into the alveoli.

18. Most of the oxygen that is transported from the lungs to the tissue spaces is transported (a) as a dissolved molecule in the plasma, (b) as oxyhemoglobin, (c) combined with hemoglobin as carbaminohemoglobin, (d) as carboxyhemoglobin.

19. The affinity of oxygen and hemoglobin decreases when (a) hydrogen ion concentration decreases, (b) carbon dioxide levels increase, (c) temperature decreases, (d) oxygen levels increase.

20. Loading of oxygen increases when the (a) intra-alveolar partial pressure of oxygen is high, (b) affinity between oxygen and hemoglobin decreases, (c) temperature increases, (d) hydrogen ion concentration increases.

21. More than two thirds of the carbon dioxide transported in the blood is (a) dissolved in plasma, (b) bound to hemoglobin, (c) attached to carbonic anhydrase, (d) in the form of bicarbonate ions in the plasma.

22. Conditions that favor the release of carbon dioxide from hemoglobin and bicarbonate ions include (a) increased oxygen and increased temperature, (b) increased temperature and increased carbon dioxide, (c) increased pH and decreased temperature, (d) decreased oxygen and increased hydrogen ion concentration.

23. The respiratory center in the brain includes neurons in the (a) medulla oblongata and the pons, (b) thalamus and pons, (c) midbrain and thalamus, (d) hypothalamus and medulla oblongata.

24. Chemoreceptors in the central nervous system stimulate inspiration when they detect (a) low oxygen levels, (b) low hydrogen ion and high carbon dioxide levels, (c) increased hydrogen ion and increased carbon dioxide levels, (d) increased hydrogen ion and decreased carbon dioxide levels.

25. Although low oxygen levels usually are not a strong stimulus for breathing, receptors that are sensitive to oxygen concentration are located (a) in the cerebrum and hypothalamus, (b) pons and medulla oblongata, (c) aortic and carotid bodies, (d) carotid bodies and pons.

A STEP BEYOND

Go a step beyond the ordinary and learn more about a topic that is related to this chapter but not discussed in detail in the textbook. Select one of the following topics, or one suggested by your instructor, and write a brief paper (250 words minimum), create a poster, or develop a short presentation (approximately 4 to 5 minutes) that focuses on your selection. Suggested topics for this chapter include the following:

1. Describe the cause and pathogenesis of asthma.

2. Describe the cause, pathogenesis, and treatment of cystic fibrosis. Learn about summer camps for children with cystic fibrosis.

3. Investigate how Henry's law of gases relates to deep sea divers and a condition called the *bends*.

4. Whenever combustible fuels, such as coal, gas, or oil are used, there is a risk of carbon monoxide poisoning. Learn about carbon monoxide poisoning. What characteristics of carbon monoxide make it a threat? How can it be prevented? What are the signs and symptoms? What is the treatment?

Word Scramble

Determine the word that fits each definition, and then write the word in the spaces below the definition, one letter per space. The letters in the boxes form a scrambled word or words. Unscramble the letters to create a word that matches the final definition in each section.

1. External nares

2. Opening between the true vocal cords

3. Primary respiratory muscle

4. Account for 70% of carbon dioxide transport

5. Instrument used to measure lung volumes

Letters to use for final word: _____

Final definition: Accounts for 23% of carbon dioxide transport

_____

6. Breathing

7. Throat

8. Most inferior laryngeal cartilage

9. Tiny air sacs in the lungs.

Letters to use for final word: _____

Final definition: Equals TV + IRV + ERV

_____

16 Digestive System

LEARNING EXERCISES

Overview and Functions of the Digestive System
Write the terms that are described by the phrases about the functions of the digestive system.

1. _____ Process of breaking large food particles into smaller ones

2. _____ Uses water to break down large molecules into smaller ones

3. _____ Breaks down complex nonabsorbable molecules into simple usable molecules

4. _____ Swallowing

5. _____ Movements that propel food through the digestive tract

6. _____ Process by which simple molecules from chemical digestion pass through the cell membranes into the blood

7. _____ Removal of indigestible wastes through the anus

General Structure of the Digestive Tract
Match the following descriptions with the correct layer of the digestive tract.

A. mucosa   B. muscular layer   C. submucosa   D. serosa

8. _____ Innermost layer of the digestive tract wall

9. _____ Contains blood and lymphatic vessels embedded in loose connective tissue

10. _____ Responsible for most movements of the digestive tract

11. _____ Consists of simple columnar epithelium in the stomach and intestines

12. _____ Contains inner circular and outer longitudinal layers

13. _____ Contains Meissner's plexus of autonomic nerve fibers

14. _____ Contains the myenteric plexus of autonomic nerve fibers

Components of the Digestive Tract
1. Write the terms that match the phrases about the oral cavity.

A. _____ Primary muscle in the cheek

B. _____ Separates oral cavity from nasal cavity

C. _____ Projection at the posterior end of the soft palate

223

D. _____ Masses of lymphoid tissue at back of tongue

E. _____ Projections on surface of the tongue

F. _____ Teeth with sharp edges for biting

G. _____ Teeth with points for grasping and tearing

H. _____ Largest salivary glands

I. _____ Glands along the medial surface of mandible

J. _____ Enzyme found in saliva

K. _____ Functions of saliva (4)

_____

_____

_____

2. Write the terms that match the phrases about the pharynx and esophagus.

A. _____ Opening from the oral cavity into the pharynx

B. _____ Most superior region of the pharynx

C. _____ Region that contains the pharyngeal tonsils

D. _____ Region that contains the palatine tonsils

E. _____ Keeps food from entering the nasopharynx

F. _____ Keeps food from entering the laryngopharynx

G. _____ Tube between the pharynx and stomach

H. _____ Opening in diaphragm for esophagus

I. _____ Sphincter between the esophagus and stomach

3. Write the terms that match the phrases about the stomach and its secretions.

A. _____ Acid in gastric juice

B. _____ Hormone secreted by gastric mucosa

C. _____ Enzyme in gastric juice

D. _____ Semifluid mixture of food and gastric juice

E. _____ Function of intrinsic factor

F. _____ Factors that influence stomach emptying (2)

_____

Match the events in the regulation of gastric secretions with the phase in which they occur.

A. cephalic phase   B. gastric phase   C. intestinal phase

4. _____   Triggered by the passage of chyme into the small intestine

5. _____   Begins with thoughts of food

6. _____   Begins when food reaches stomach

7. _____   Inhibits gastric secretions

8. _____   Involves distention of the stomach wall

9. Write the terms that match the phrases about the small intestine and its secretions.

A. _____ Region adjacent to the stomach

B. _____ Features that increase the surface area (3)

_____

_____

C. _____ Lymph capillary in a villus

D. _____ Has mucous glands in the submucosa

E. _____ Region with most goblet cells

F. _____ Activates a pancreatic enzyme

G. _____ Stimulates the release of bile from gallbladder

H. _____ Stimulates pancreatic release of bicarbonate

I. _____ Acts on neutral fats

J. _____ Stimulates pancreatic digestive enzymes

K. _____ Most important factor for regulating secretions of the small intestine

10. What are the two main functions of the large intestine?

   A. _____

   B. _____

11. Match the descriptive phrases with the correct terms.

   A. _____ Where the small intestine enters the large intestine

   B. _____ Three bands of longitudinal muscle in the large intestine

   C. _____ Pieces of fat-filled connective tissue attached to the colon

   D. _____ Blind pouch that extends inferiorly from entrance of the ileum

   E. _____ Portion of the large intestine on the right side

   F. _____ Right colonic flexure

   G. _____ Left colonic flexure

   H. _____ Portion of the large intestine between the two colonic flexures

   I. _____ Portion of the large intestine on the left side

   J. _____ S-shaped curve across the pelvic brim

   K. _____ Portion that follows the curvature of the sacrum

   L. _____ Terminal opening of the digestive tract

   M. _____ Series of pouches in the large intestine

   1. anus
   2. ascending colon
   3. cecum
   4. descending colon
   5. epiploic appendages
   6. haustra
   7. hepatic flexure
   8. ileocecal junction
   9. rectum
   10. sigmoid colon
   11. splenic flexure
   12. teniae coli
   13. transverse colon

12. Match each of the following descriptions with the appropriate structure. Each description has only one response. Responses are to be used only once, and not all responses will be used.

   A. _____ Opening from the oral cavity into the pharynx

   B. _____ Portion of the stomach that is superior to the entrance of the esophagus

   C. _____ Circular band of muscle at the exit from the stomach

   D. _____ Circular folds of mucosa in the small intestine

   E. _____ Circular band of muscle between the esophagus and stomach

   F. _____ Curve between the ascending colon and the transverse colon

   G. _____ Longitudinal folds of mucosa in the stomach

   H. _____ Longitudinal muscle bands in the large intestine

   I. _____ Shortest part of the small intestine

   J. _____ Circular band of muscle between the small intestine and large intestine

   1. duodenum
   2. fauces
   3. fundus
   4. haustra
   5. hepatic flexure
   6. ileocecal sphincter
   7. ileum
   8. jejunum
   9. lower esophageal sphincter
   10. plicae circulares
   11. pyloric sphincter
   12. pylorus
   13. rugae
   14. splenic flexure
   15. teniae coli

Accessory Organs of Digestion

1. Write the terms that match the phrases about the liver.

A. _____ Attaches the liver to the anterior abdominal wall

B. _____ Region between the ligamentum venosum and inferior vena cava

C. _____ Region between the ligamentum teres and gallbladder

D. _____ Functional unit of the liver

E. _____ Venous channels between hepatocytes

F. _____ Vessel that carries oxygen-rich blood to the liver

G. _____ Vessel that carries nutrient-rich blood to the liver

H. _____ Vessel that carries blood away from the liver

I. _____ Secretory product of the liver

J. _____ Principal bile pigment

K. _____ Function of bile salts

L. _____ Area of bile storage

M. _____ Duct that attaches gallbladder to liver

N. _____ Stimulates the release of bile from the gallbladder

O. _____ Duct that enters the duodenum

P. _____ Components of a portal triad (3)

_____

_____

2. Write the terms that match the phrases about the pancreas.

A. _____ Endocrine portion of the pancreas

B. _____ Exocrine portion of the pancreas

C. _____ Carries pancreatic enzymes to the duodenum

D. _____ Pancreatic enzyme that acts on starch

E. _____ Pancreatic enzyme that acts on proteins

F. _____ Breaks fats into fatty acids and monoglycerides

G. _____ Hormones that regulate pancreatic secretions (2)

_____

Chemical Digestion

1. Complete the following table about enzymes and their role in digestion.

Enzyme	Source	Digestive Action
	Salivary glands/pancreas	Complex carbohydrates to disaccharides
		Maltose to glucose
Sucrase		
		Lactose to glucose and galactose
	Stomach	Proteins to polypeptides
Trypsin		Proteins to polypeptides
		Peptides to amino acids
		Fats to fatty acids and monoglycerides

2. What are the three monosaccharides that are the end products of carbohydrate digestion?

_____

3. What are the end products of protein digestion?

_____

4. What are the two primary end products of lipid digestion?

_____

Absorption

1. Write the terms that match the phrases about the absorption of nutrients.

A. _____ Villus vessel that absorbs amino acids and simple sugars

B. _____ Villus vessel that absorbs triglycerides

C. _____ Fatty acids coated with bile salts

D. _____ Triglycerides combined with proteins

E. _____ Mixture of lymph and digested fats

2. Write the transport process that is responsible for each of the following movements.

A. _____ Glucose from lumen of small intestine into villus cells

B. _____ Fructose from lumen of small intestine into villus cells

C. _____ Water throughout the length of the digestive tract

D. _____ Most nutrients from villus cells to capillaries and lacteals

3. The following six items are end products of digestion. Indicate whether each is a product of carbohydrate (C), protein (P), or fat (F) digestion and whether it is absorbed by the blood capillaries (B) or lacteals (L) of the villi. Each end product should be designated by a C, P, or an F and by a B or an L.

C, P, F	B or L	
		Glucose
		Amino acids
		Monoglycerides
		Fructose
		Fatty acids
		Galactose

LABELING & COLORING EXERCISES

Identify the parts of the digestive system by matching the letters from Figure 16-1 with the terms on the left. Place an asterisk (*) by the accessory organs.

1. _____   Esophagus
2. _____   Gallbladder
3. _____   Large intestine
4. _____   Liver
5. _____   Mouth
6. _____   Pancreas
7. _____   Pharynx
8. _____   Salivary gland
9. _____   Small intestine
10. _____   Stomach

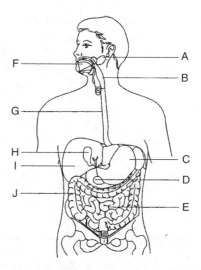

Figure 16-1   Organs of the digestive system.

Identify the parts of a tooth by matching the letters from Figure 16-2 with the correct terms.

11. _____   Alveolar process
12. _____   Apical foramen
13. _____   Cementum
14. _____   Dentin
15. _____   Enamel
16. _____   Gingiva
17. _____   Pulp cavity
18. _____   Root canal

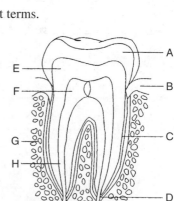

Figure 16-2   Structure of a tooth.

229

Identify the regions of the stomach by matching the letters from Figure 16-3 with the correct terms. Outline the greater curvature in red and the lesser curvature in blue.

19. _____ Body

20. _____ Cardiac region

21. _____ Duodenum

22. _____ Fundus

23. _____ Lower esophageal sphincter

24. _____ Pyloric sphincter

25. _____ Pylorus

26. _____ Rugae

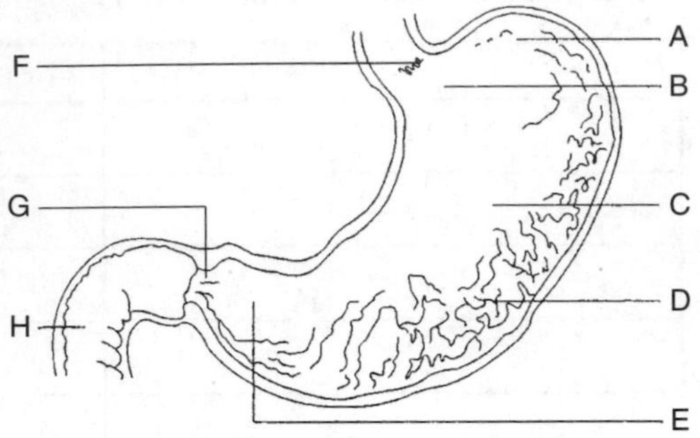

Figure 16-3 Features of the stomach

REVIEW QUESTIONS

1. Name, in sequence, the regions of the digestive tract.

_____   _____

_____   _____

_____   _____

2. What five activities of the digestive system prepare nutrients for use by the body?

_____

_____

_____

_____

_____

3. Name, in sequence starting with the innermost, the four layers in the wall of the digestive tract.

_____   _____

_____   _____

4. What are the submucosal (Meissner's) plexus and myenteric (Auerbach's) plexus?

A. _____

B. _____

5. Where are the hard and soft palates located? What is the difference in structure between them?

_____

_____

_____

6. What type of muscle makes up the substance of the tongue?

_____

7. What is another name for *primary teeth?* How many teeth are in this set?

_____

_____

8. What four types of teeth, based on shape, are found in the secondary teeth?

_____

_____

9. What substance covers the crown of a tooth?

_____

10. Where is the largest salivary gland located?

_____

_____

11. What enzyme is found in saliva?

_____

12. What is the fauces?

_____

_____

13. Where is the lower esophageal sphincter located? What is another name for this structure?

_____

_____

14. What are the four regions of the stomach?

_____   _____

_____   _____

15. How does the muscular layer of the stomach differ from that in other regions of the digestive tract?

_____

_____

16. Name the type of cell that produces (a) pepsinogen, (b) hydrochloric acid, (c) gastrin, (d) intrinsic factor.

_____   _____

_____   _____

17. What hormone and what cranial nerve are involved in regulating gastric juice secretion?

_____

18. What sphincter relaxes to allow chyme to pass from the stomach into the small intestine?

_____

19. What three features of the small intestine increase its absorptive surface area?

_____

20. Chyme first enters what part of the small intestine? Secretions from what two glands also enter this region?

_____

21. Which region of the small intestine has (a) the longest villi, (b) an opening for the cystic duct, (c) the most goblet cells, (d) an opening for the pancreatic duct, (e) mucous glands in the submucosa?

_____

_____

_____

_____

22. What is the function of (a) maltase, (b) peptidase, (c) secretin, (d) enterokinase, (e) cholecystokinin?

_____

_____

_____

_____

_____

23. What is the most important factor that regulates the secretion of enzymes and hormones in the small intestine?

_____

24. What are teniae coli, haustra, and epiploic appendages?

_____

_____

_____

25. Between which two parts of the large intestine is the hepatic flexure located? Splenic flexure?

_____

_____

26. Which anal sphincter is controlled voluntarily?

_____

27. What are two functions of the large intestine?

_____

_____

28. What ligament attaches the anterior surface of the liver to the anterior abdominal wall?

_____

29. Name three boundaries of the caudate lobe of the liver.

_____

_____

_____

30. What are the components of a portal triad?

_____

_____

_____

31. What two blood vessels bring blood to the liver sinusoids?

_____

32. What function of the liver is specifically related to digestion?

_____

33. What two substances are excreted in the bile?

_____

34. What hormone stimulates the gallbladder to contract?

_____

35. Where is the pancreas located?

_____

_____

36. What cells in the pancreas secrete enzymes that are important in digestion?

_____

37. What is the function of (a) amylase, (b) trypsin, (c) peptidase, (d) lipase?

_____

_____

_____

_____

38. Use the terms *secretin* and *cholecystokinin* in a description of the regulation of pancreatic secretion.

_____

_____

_____

_____

39. What are the end products of carbohydrate digestion?

_____

40. Name two enzymes that are involved in the digestion of proteins into peptides.

_____

_____

41. What are the end products of lipid digestion?

_____

_____

42. What structures absorb simple sugars and amino acids in the small intestine? What structures absorb fatty acids and monoglycerides?

_____

_____

_____

FUNCTIONAL RELATIONSHIPS

It is important to remember that no system in the body works alone. It takes the interaction of all systems to maintain homeostasis. The following exercises reinforce the concept that all systems work together to maintain the health and wellbeing of other systems and the individual.

Match the system on the right with what it provides for the digestive system on the left. Use the functional relationships page in your concepts textbook as a resource.

1. _____ Provides vitamin D for absorption of calcium in intestine

2. _____ Provides attachment for muscles of mastication

3. _____ Provides action for chewing, swallowing, peristalsis, and defecation

4. _____ Controls motility and glandular activity of digestive tract

5. _____ Influences secretion of gallbladder and pancreas

6. _____ Transports nutrients and delivers hormones

7. _____ Absorbs fats and fat-soluble vitamins from digestive tract

8. _____ Maintains pH for enzyme action

9. _____ Excretes metabolic wastes produced by liver

10. _____ Steroids affect metabolic rate

A. Cardiovascular

B. Endocrine

C. Integumentary

D. Lymphatic

E. Muscular

F. Nervous

G. Reproductive

H. Respiratory

I. Skeletal

J. Urinary

For each of the following systems, write what the digestive system provides for it.

11. Cardiovascular _____

_____

12. Skeletal _____

13. Reproductive _____

_____

14. Endocrine _____

15. Lymphatic _____

_____

16. Muscular _____

_____

17. Nervous _____

_____

18. Respiratory _____

19. Urinary _____

20. Integumentary _____

235

REPRESENTATIVE DISORDERS

Match the disorder of the digestive system on the right with its description of the left.

1. _____ A deterioration of the mucosa of the esophagus, stomach, or duodenum

2. _____ Inflammation of the liver

3. _____ Chronic liver disease marked by degeneration of liver cells

4. _____ Difficulty in swallowing

5. _____ Formation of gallstones

6. _____ Inflammation of the stomach lining

7. _____ Protrusion of a structure through an opening in the diaphragm

8. _____ Inflammation of the gallbladder

9. _____ Disorder caused by lack of insulin

10. _____ Chronic, relapsing inflammation of the intestinal tract

A. Cholecystitis

B. Cholelithiasis

C. Cirrhosis

D. Crohn disease

E. Diabetes mellitus

F. Dysphagia

G. Gastritis

H. Hepatitis

I. Hiatal hernia

J. Peptic ulcers

VOCABULARY PRACTICE

Match the definitions on the left with the correct clinical term from the column on the right by placing the corresponding letter in the space before the definition. Not all terms will be used.

1. _____ Folds in the stomach mucosa

2. _____ Semifluid mixture of food and gastric juice that enters the small intestine

3. _____ Twisting of the bowel that causes an obstruction

4. _____ An emotional disorder characterized by binge eating

5. _____ Drugs that increase the rate of fecal movement through the colon

6. _____ Folds in the mucosa and submucosa of the small intestine

7. _____ Blood in the vomit

8. _____ Heartburn; regurgitation of stomach acid into the esophagus

9. _____ Drugs that reduce peristalsis in the intestines

10. _____ Accumulation of serous fluid in the peritoneal cavity

A. Anorexia

B. Antidiarrheals

C. Ascites

D. Bulimia

E. Chyle

F. Chyme

G. Hematemesis

H. Laxatives

I. Plicae circulares

J. Pyrosis

K. Rugae

L. Volvulus

11. Write the meaning of the following abbreviations.

A. _____ GERD

B. _____ NPO

C. _____ GI

D. _____ GB

E. _____ FOBT

F. _____ CLD

G. _____ IBD

H. _____ LES

I. _____ TPN

J. _____ PUD

12. Spelling is important in scientific and medical applications because only one or two incorrect letters can change the meaning. Circle the correctly spelled word for each of the following pairs.

    A. esophageal   esophogeal

    B. postpandial   postprandial

    C. glosopharyngeal   glossopharyngeal

    D. masetter   masseter

    E. monoglycerides   monoglyserides

13. Write the meaning of the underlined portion of each word on the line preceding the word.

    A. _____ _____ cholecystectomy

    B. _____ enteropathy

    C. _____ cholecystectomy

    D. _____ gingivitis

    E. _____ hepatomegaly

    F. _____ anorexia

    G. _____ sialadenectomy

    H. _____ sialadenectomy

    I. ___ _____ sialadenectomy

    J. _____ hematemesis

14. For each of the following words, underline the word part that corresponds to the underlined word or phrase in the definition.

    A. cheiloplasty   plastic surgery of the lip

    B. glossopathy   any disease of the tongue

    C. dentalgia   tooth pain

    D. biliary   pertaining to bile

    E. gastralgia   pain in the stomach

    F. peristalsis   wavelike contractions of the digestive tube

    G. hematochezia   blood in the feces

    H. linguopapillitis   inflammation of the papillae on the tongue

    I. postprandial   after a meal

    J. gingivectomy   surgical excision of diseased tissue of the gums

15. Answer the following questions.

   A. Dee Jeston had a salivary gland removed by surgery. What is the medical term for this procedure?

   _____

   B. Janie Student's baby was vomiting almost continuously. Use your knowledge of word parts to write the medical term for this condition of excessive vomiting.

   _____

   C. Drew Deenum complained of pain in and around the rectum and anus. Use your knowledge of word parts to write the medical term for this condition.

   _____

TESTING COMPREHENSION

Multiple choice: Select the best response.

1. Which of the following terms refers to chemical digestion? (a) mastication, (b) hydrolysis, (c) peristalsis, (d) deglutition.

2. Starting from the inside, or lumen, the sequence of layers in the wall of the gastrointestinal tract is (a) serosa, mucosa, submucosa, muscular; (b) mucosa, submucosa, inner longitudinal muscle, outer circular muscle; (c) serosa, muscular, submucosa, mucosa; (d) mucosa, submucosa, muscular, serosa.

3. Nerve plexuses for autonomic control of the gastrointestinal tract are located in the (a) submucosa and muscular layers, (b) mucosa and submucosa layers, (c) muscular and serosa layers, (d) mucosa and serosa layers.

4. In a normal set of permanent teeth, how many teeth are in the right upper jaw? (a) 5, (b) 8, (c) 12, (d) 16.

5. The teeth that are sharp and pointed for grasping and tearing food are the (a) incisors, (b) canines, (c) bicuspids, (d) molars.

6. The substance that surrounds the pulp cavity and forms the bulk of the tooth is the (a) crown, (d) enamel, (c) dentin, (d) cementum.

7. The largest salivary glands are the (a) sublingual, (b) submandibular, (c) submaxillary, (d) parotid.

8. The digestive enzyme in saliva is (a) amylase, (b) lipase, (c) sucrase, (d) maltase.

9. The esophagus (a) secretes enzymes for the digestion of starch, (b) secretes intrinsic factor, (c) is a tube that is posterior to the trachea, (d) has an opening called the fauces.

10. Which of the following is true about the stomach? (a) it functions in the digestion of fats, (b) its wall has three layers of muscle, (c) the mucosa has folds called plicae circulares, (d) villi in the mucosa facilitate absorption.

11. The region of the stomach around the lower esophageal sphincter is the (a) pylorus, (b) body, (c) fundus, (d) cardiac region.

12. Regarding gastric secretions, (a) parietal cells secrete intrinsic factor, (b) chief cells secrete hydrochloric acid, (c) endocrine cells secrete pepsinogen, (d) goblet cells secrete gastrin.

13. The gastric phase of stomach activity begins when (a) a person sees or smells food, (b) a person tastes and chews food, (c) chyme passes through the pyloric sphincter, (d) food passes through the lower esophageal sphincter.

14. The shortest portion of the small intestine is the (a) cecum, (b) ileum, (c) jejunum, (d) duodenum.

15. Intestinal glands secrete (a) intrinsic factor, (b) maltase, (c) pepsinogen, (d) gastrin.

238

16. Features of the large intestine include (a) haustra and teniae coli, (b) plicae circulares and brush border, (c) rugae and villi, (d) goblet cells and microvilli.

17. The portion of the colon that is on the left side is the (c) cecum, (b) ascending colon, (c) hepatic flexure, (d) descending colon.

18. Exocrine secretions from the pancreas enter the (a) stomach, (b) duodenum, (c) jejunum, (d) ileum.

19. The liver is attached to the anterior abdominal wall by the (a) falciform ligament, (b) ligamentum teres, (c) ligamentum venosum, (d) greater omentum.

20. Which of the following in *not* correct about bile? (a) it is stored in the gallbladder, (b) it helps to neutralize the acidity of chyme, (c) it contains lipase for the digestion of fats, (c) it contains bile pigments from the breakdown of red blood cells (RBCs).

21. Which of the following is *not* a function of the liver? (a) synthesizes fibrinogen and clotting factors, (b) removes bacteria and damaged RBCs from the blood, (c) synthesizes bile salts from cholesterol, (d) produces secretin and cholecystokinin.

22. The gallbladder is attached to the liver by the (a) cystic duct, (b) hepatic duct, (c) common bile duct, (d) hepatopancreatic duct.

23. Exocrine secretions from the pancreas include (a) insulin and lipase, (b) trypsin and glucagon, (c) amylase and enterokinase, (d) trypsinogen and lipase.

24. Most of the digestion of food into molecules that can be absorbed occurs in the (a) stomach, (b) small intestine, (c) large intestine, (d) liver.

25. Most of the absorption of molecules from the cells of the villi into the blood capillaries and lacteals is by the process of (a) diffusion, (b) osmosis, (c) active transport, (d) filtration.

A STEP BEYOND

Go a step beyond the ordinary and learn more about a topic that is related to this chapter but not discussed in detail in the textbook. Select one of the following topics, or one suggested by your instructor, and write a brief paper (250 words minimum), create a poster, or develop a short presentation (approximately 4 to 5 minutes) that focuses on your selection. Suggested topics for this chapter include the following:

1. *Lactose intolerance*. What is it? What populations are most susceptible? How can it be treated? What are some of the problems associated with being lactose intolerant?
2. *Anorexia and bulimia*. What are they? Compare the two disorders. What are the risks associated with them? How can they be treated?
3. *Cirrhosis of the liver*. What is cirrhosis of the liver? Describe its causes and pathogenesis. How does alcoholism relate to liver cirrhosis? What are the effects of the disease? How can it be avoided?
4. *Tobacco and cancer of the mouth, throat, and esophagus*. Is there a relationship between the use of tobacco products and cancer of the digestive tract? What are the risks and treatments? What are the specific carcinogenic agents?
5. *Dental caries*. What is the pathogenesis of tooth decay? Is there a relationship between dental hygiene and general health? Will flossing your teeth help you live longer?

FUN & GAMES

Word Scramble

Determine the word that fits each definition, and then write the word in the spaces across from the definition, one letter per space. The letters in the boxes form a scrambled word or words. Unscramble the letters to create a word that matches the final definition in each section.

1. Peritoneum associated with the small intestine

2. Receives food from the esophagus

3. Cells that secrete hydrochloric acid

4. Hormone that stimulates the release of bile

[grid of boxes with circles for letters]

Letters to use for final word: _____

Final definition: Form in which fatty acids are absorbed

_____

5. Tube between the pharynx and stomach

[grid of boxes with circles]

6. Main muscle in the cheek

[grid of boxes with circles]

7. Tiny hairlike extension on the villi

[grid of boxes with circles]

8. Main portion of the stomach

[grid of boxes with circles]

Letters to use for final word: _____

Final definition: Rumbling noise caused by propulsion of gas through the intestines

_____

17 Metabolism and Nutrition

Metabolism of Absorbed Nutrients

1. Write the terms that match the given definitions.

A. _____ Total of all chemical reactions in the body

B. _____ Chemical reactions within cells to produce energy

C. _____ Substances that speed up physiologic reactions

D. _____ Acquisition and utilization of nutrients

Match the following terms with the correct definitions or descriptive phrases.

A. acetyl CoA	F. deamination	K. glycogenolysis
B. aerobic	G. gluconeogenesis	L. glycolysis
C. anaerobic	H. glucose	M. lactic acid
D. beta oxidation	I. glycogen	N. lipogenesis
E. cytoplasm	J. glycogenesis	O. mitochondria

2. _____ Most important simple sugar in cellular metabolism

3. _____ Term that means oxygen is not required

4. _____ Reactions in which glucose is split into two molecules of pyruvic acid

5. _____ Fate of pyruvic acid in absence of oxygen

6. _____ Term that means oxygen is required

7. _____ Molecule that enters the citric acid cycle

8. _____ Storage form of glucose

9. _____ Location of glycolysis reactions

10. _____ Location of citric acid cycle reactions

11. _____ Conversion of glucose to glycogen

12. _____ Conversion of glucose to fat

13. _____ Conversion of glycogen into glucose

14. _____ Conversion of noncarbohydrates to glucose

15. _____ Principal reaction that prepares amino acids for use as an energy source

16. _____ Reactions that convert fatty acids to acetyl CoA

17. State six uses of the proteins that are synthesized in the body. Do not include their possible use as an energy source.

A. _____

B. _____

C. _____

D. _____

E. _____

F. _____

18. What are the two key molecules in the interconversion of carbohydrates, proteins, and fats?

_____   _____

19. Define or explain what is meant by the nutritional calorie or kilocalorie.

_____

_____

20. List the three uses of energy in the body. Draw a circle around the one that accounts for most of the energy used. Place an asterisk (*) by the one that can be controlled voluntarily.

A. _____

B. _____

C. _____

Body Temperature

Match the following terms with the correct definitions or descriptive phrases about body temperature.

A. blood   F. hypothalamus

B. constriction of vessels in skin   G. perspiration

C. core temperature   H. radiation

D. epinephrine   I. shell temperature

E. heat   J. shivering

1. _____ By-product of cellular metabolism

2. _____ Location of the body's thermostat

3. _____ Temperature of internal organs

4. _____ Heat-producing hormone

5. _____ Distributes heat through the body

6. _____ Methods of increasing body heat (2)

   _____

7. _____ Methods of releasing body heat (2)

   _____

8. _____ Temperature at the body surface

Basic Elements of Nutrition

1. Indicate whether each of the following most closely applies to carbohydrates, lipids, or proteins. Use C = carbohydrates, L = lipids, and P = proteins.

   A. _____ Primary energy source

   B. _____ Regulate body processes

   C. _____ Major component of cell membranes

   D. _____ Transport vitamins A, D, E, K

   E. _____ Add bulk to the diet

   F. _____ Fatty acids

   G. _____ Provide insulation and protection

   H. _____ Provide structure

   I. _____ Glucose

   J. _____ Concentrated energy

   K. _____ Fiber

   L. _____ Hormones, enzymes

   M. _____ Steroids

   N. _____ Glycogen

   O. _____ Triglycerides

   P. _____ Amino acids

2. How many calories are in each of the following?

   A. _____ 1 g pure carbohydrate

   B. _____ 1 g pure protein

   C. _____ 1 g pure fat

   D. _____ 5 g carbohydrate

   E. _____ 4 g protein

   F. _____ 3 g fat

3. Complete the following paragraph by writing the correct words in the blanks.

   Amino acids that cannot be synthesized in the body and must be supplied in the diet are called _____

   amino acids. A protein that contains all these amino acids is called a _____

   protein. Other proteins, called *incomplete proteins*, should be eaten in combinations to provide all the

   _____ amino acids.

4. Complete the following paragraph by writing the correct words in the blanks.

   The American Heart Association recommends that no more than _____ of the daily

   calorie intake should be in the form of fats. Further, it recommends a reduction in the amount of saturated fats in the

   diet. In general, foods that are high in saturated fats are also high in _____. Cholesterol

   intake should be limited to less than _____ per day.

243

5. Classify the following vitamins as being either water soluble or fat soluble. Use W for water soluble and F for fat soluble.

A. _____ Thiamine   C. _____ Vitamin A   E. _____ Vitamin D

B. _____ Niacin   D. _____ Vitamin C   F. _____ Riboflavin

6. Indicate whether each of the following most closely applies to uses of vitamins, minerals, or water in the body. Use V = vitamins, M = minerals, and W = water.

A. _____ Medium for chemical reactions   D. _____ Incorporated into bones and teeth

B. _____ Release energy from nutrients   E. _____ Maintenance of body temperature

C. _____ Nucleic acid synthesis   F. _____ Regulation of body fluid levels

REVIEW QUESTIONS

1. What is the relationship between metabolism and nutrition?

_____

_____

_____

2. What group of reactions releases chemical energy in the cell, and what molecule represents this chemical energy?

_____

_____

3. Where in the cell does glycolysis take place and what are the end products?

_____

_____

4. What happens to pyruvic acid in the aerobic phase of cellular respiration, and where does this occur?

_____

_____

5. How do glycogenesis and glycogenolysis help maintain a constant blood glucose lever?

_____

_____

_____

6. What is the primary purpose of amino acids in the body?

_____

7. What type of reaction prepares amino acids so they can be used as a source of energy?

_____

8. What type of chemical reaction is involved in the catabolism of fatty acids? What is the end product of this process?

_____

_____

9. What are the two key molecules in gluconeogenesis?

_____

10. What is the difference between basal metabolic rate and total metabolic rate?

_____

_____

11. Which component of energy expenditure can be controlled voluntarily?

_____

12. Compare the amounts of energy that can be obtained from 1 g of carbohydrate, protein, and fat.

_____

_____

_____

13. What are homeotherms?

_____

14. Which is greater, core temperature or shell temperature?

_____

15. What is the main source of heat to maintain core temperature?

_____

16. What accounts for most of the heat loss from the body?

_____

17. Where is the body's thermostat located?

_____

18. What is the form in which carbohydrate is carried in the blood?

_____

19. Give a common food source for (a) fructose, (b) sucrose; (c) lactose; (d) maltose.

_____   _____

_____   _____

245

20. Starch and fiber are derived from plant sources. What is their difference in terms of utilization?

_____

_____

21. In what ways do proteins help regulate body processes?

_____

_____

22. Why are certain amino acids termed *essential*?

_____

_____

23. What is lacking in an incomplete protein?

_____

24. What category of nutrients represents a concentrated energy source?

_____

25. What is the American Heart Association's recommendation regarding dietary intake of saturated fats? What common food sources are high in saturated fats?

_____

_____

26. What vitamins require fats for absorption and utilization?

_____

_____

27. Why are vitamins and minerals necessary in the diet?

_____

_____

_____

28. What are the primary food sources of minerals?

_____

29. Why is water essential to good health?

_____

_____

VOCABULARY PRACTICE

Match the definitions on the left with the correct clinical term from the column on the right by placing the corresponding letter in the space before the definition. Not all terms will be used.

1. _____ Production of heat in response to food intake

2. _____ Amount of energy necessary to maintain life at a minimal level

3. _____ Intravenous approach to nutrition

4. _____ Yellow skin color caused by excessive bilirubin

5. _____ A state of poor nourishment

6. _____ Temperature of internal organs

7. _____ Nutrients enter some region of the GI tract

8. _____ Deficiency of protein and calorie intake

9. _____ Absence of HCl in gastric secretions

10. _____ Inadequate food intake

A. Achlorhydria
B. Basal metabolic rate
C. Core temperature
D. Enteral nutrition
E. Jaundice
F. Kwashiorkor
G. Malnutrition
H. Marasmus
I. Parenteral nutrition
J. Shell temperature
K. Thermogenesis
L. Undernutrition

11. Write the meaning of the following abbreviations.

A. _____ BBT

B. _____ BMR

C. _____ HDL

D. _____ TPN

E. _____ BMI

F. _____ TPR

G. _____ D/W

H. _____ MNT

I. _____ PPBS

J. _____ FUO

12. Spelling is important in scientific and medical applications because only one or two incorrect letters can change the meaning. Circle the correctly spelled word for each of the following pairs.

A. anairobic   anaerobic

B. asetyl-CoA   acetyl-CoA

C. triglycerides   triglyserides

D. homeotherm   homiotherm

E. glucogenolysis   glycogenolysis

13. Write the meaning of the underlined portion of each word on the line preceding the word.

A. _____ glyco<u>gen</u>esis

B. _____ nutri<u>tion</u>

C. _____ dys<u>peps</u>ia

D. _____ <u>ana</u>bolism

E. _____ glyco<u>lys</u>is

F. _____ <u>cata</u>bolism

G. _____ <u>mal</u>nutrition

H. _____ py<u>ro</u>genic

I. _____ <u>vita</u>min

J. _____ gluco<u>neo</u>genesis

14. Wally O. Beese went to his primary care physician (PCP) for a follow-up after having some blood work done. The PCP explained that he was at risk for CAD because his blood showed elevated levels of "bad" cholesterol. He also suggested that Wally try to lose weight by increasing his metabolic rate and by reducing his intake of fatty foods such as French fries, butter, and potato chips.

A. What is CAD?

_____

B. What is the medical term for "bad" cholesterol?

_____

C. Why does "bad" cholesterol increase the risk of CAD?

_____

_____

D. What part of total metabolic rate can be voluntarily controlled?

_____

E. Why do fats cause more weight gain than an equal quantity of carbohydrates?

_____

_____

TESTING COMPREHENSION

Multiple choice: Select the best response.

1. Which one of the following refers to anabolism? (a) releases energy, (b) cellular respiration, (c) dehydration synthesis, (d) breaks large molecules into smaller ones.

2. The acquisition and assimilation of foods is called (a) metabolism, (b) nutrition, (c) diet, (d) alimentation.

3. The first series of reactions in the catabolism of glucose (a) requires oxygen, (b) occurs in the mitochondria, (c) produces acetyl CoA, (d) is called glycolysis.

4. The end product of glycolysis is (a) pyruvic acid, (b) acetyl CoA, (c) citric acid, (d) glycogen.

5. Which of the following is *not* correct about the citric acid cycle? (a) it requires oxygen, (b) it occurs in the mitochondria, (c) it produces adenosine triphosphate (ATP), (d) it converts acetyl CoA to pyruvic acid.

6. The carbohydrate molecule that is the storage form of glucose in humans is (a) glycogen, (b) starch, (c) triglyceride, (d) maltose.

7. When proteins are used as an energy source, the principal reaction that prepares the amino acids for use as energy is (a) gluconeogenesis, (b) beta oxidation, (c) deamination, (d) glycolysis.

8. The process of deamination produces (a) urea, (b) ammonia, (c) acetone, (d) lactic acid.

9. Beta oxidation (a) is a reaction in protein catabolism, (b) is a step in the conversion of amino acids to glucose, (c) produces urea, (d) splits two-carbon molecules from the end of a fatty acid.

10. A gram of carbohydrate yields (a) 1 Calorie of energy, (b) 4 Calories of energy, (c) 6 Calories of energy, (d) 9 Calories of energy.

11. The greatest amount of energy is used for (a) basal metabolism, (b) physical activity, (c) thermogenesis, (d) physical activity plus thermogenesis.

12. How many grams of fat will produce the same number of nutritional calories as 9 g of carbohydrate? (a) 9 g of fat, (b) 4 g of fat, (c) 1 g of fat, (d) 2 ½ g of fat.

13. The heat loss mechanism that is responsible for the most heat loss from the body is (a) radiation, (b) conduction, (c) convection, (d) evaporation.

14. The temperature regulating system (body thermostat) is located in the (a) medulla oblongata, (b) carotid bodies, (c) hypothalamus, (d) pons.

15. In response to a cold environment, (a) the cutaneous blood vessels dilate so you feel warmer, (b) the metabolic rate decreases to conserve heat, (c) core temperature decreases before shell temperature, (d) epinephrine and norepinephrine promote heat production.

16. Which of the following is a monosaccharide? (a) sucrose, (b) fructose, (c) maltose, (d) lactose.

17. Common table sugar is (a) sucrose, (b) fructose, (c) glucose, (d) maltose.

18. Which of the following does *not* apply to dietary fiber? (a) it cannot be digested by humans, (b) it adds bulk to the diet, (c) it is commonly found in processed and refined foods, (d) it enhances the absorption of nutrients.

19. Some amino acids are called nonessential because (a) they are not necessary for protein synthesis, (b) they can be made from other amino acids in the body, (c) they can be derived from carbohydrate sources, (d) they are found in complete proteins.

249

20. Lipids (a) are not necessary in the diet, (b) function in the absorption of certain vitamins; (c) are necessary for maintaining fluid balance in the body; (d) are found only in animal products such as meat, butter, and eggs.

21. Trans fat (a) is produced by hydrogenation of unsaturated fats, (b) contains very little cholesterol, (c) is healthier to use than liquid oils, (d) contains only non-essential fatty acids.

22. Fat-soluble vitamins include (a) folic acid and niacin, (b) vitamin C and riboflavin, (c) vitamin B_{12} and vitamin K, (d) vitamin E and vitamin A.

23. The vitamin that is necessary for the synthesis of clotting factors is found in (a) milk, (b) citrus fruit, (c) fish oil, (d) green leafy vegetables.

24. The mineral that is essential for the synthesis of thyroid hormones is (a) calcium, (b) iodine, (c) sodium, (d) iron.

25. The best sources for minerals are (a) fruits and vegetables, (b) fortified milk, (c) eggs and meat, (d) cheese and water.

A STEP BEYOND

Go a step beyond the ordinary and learn more about a topic that is related to this chapter but not discussed in detail in the textbook. Select one of the following topics, or one suggested by your instructor, and write a brief paper (250 words minimum), create a poster, or develop a short presentation (approximately 4 to 5 minutes) that focuses on your selection. Suggested topics for this chapter:

1. U.S. Department of Agriculture (USDA) food pyramid. Learn about their recommended food pyramid. Keep track of everything you eat and drink, including snacks, for a minimum of 3 days. How does your dietary intake compare to the USDA food pyramid?
2. Vegetarian and vegan diets. What is the difference between these two types of diets? What are the pros and cons of these diets relative to good health? How can essential nutrients be obtained when following these diets?
3. Obesity and fitness. What is obesity? How does it differ from poor physical fitness? How is obesity measured? What health risks are associated with obesity?
4. Obesity and eating. Weight gain is primarily a matter of consuming more calories than you use. There are some physiologic factors that tend to alter the balance. Investigate physiologic factors that tend to make a person obese and what can be done to counteract these factors.

FUN & GAMES

Word Scramble

Determine the word that fits each definition, and then write the word in the spaces below the definition, one letter per space. The letters in the boxes form a scrambled word or words. Unscramble the letters to create a word that matches the final definition in each section.

1. Anaerobic catabolism of glucose

2. A complex carbohydrate

3. Warm-blooded animals

4. Storage form of glucose

Letters to use for final word: _____

Final definition: Heat production

_____

5. Building up processes that require energy

6. Most common form of lipids in the diet

7. Most important carbohydrate in cellular respiration

8. Catabolic reaction in protein metabolism

Letters to use for final word: _____

Final definition: Conversion of noncarbohydrates to glucose

_____

18 Urinary System and Body Fluids

LEARNING EXERCISES

Functions of the Urinary System

1. What are the six functions of the urinary system?

A. _____   D. _____

B. _____   E. _____

C. _____   F. _____

Components of the Urinary System

1. Name the four components of the urinary system in the sequence in which urine flows through them.

A. _____   C. _____

B. _____   D. _____

2. Write the terms that match the following phrases.

A. _____   Modified cells in the ascending limb

B. _____   Modified cells in the afferent arteriole

C. _____   Enzyme produced by juxtaglomerular cells

D. _____   Structure that monitors NaCl in the urine

E. _____   Rate of blood flow through the kidney

F. _____   Arteries located in the renal sinus

G. _____   Arteries located in the renal columns

H. _____   Branches of the arcuate arteries

I. _____   Vessel that carries blood to the glomerulus

J. _____   Capillary network around renal tubules

K. _____   Location of the interlobar vein

L. _____   Veins that join to form the renal vein

3. Write the terms that match the following phrases about the ureters, urinary bladder, and urethra.

A. _____ Transport urine from the kidney to urinary bladder

B. _____ Epithelium in the mucosa of ureters

C. _____ Temporary storage site for urine

D. _____ Folds in the mucosa of urinary bladder

E. _____ Epithelium in the mucosa of urinary bladder

F. _____ Smooth muscle in the wall of urinary bladder

G. _____ Triangular region in the floor of urinary bladder

H. _____ Muscle type forming internal urethral sphincter

I. _____ Muscle type forming external urethral sphincter

J. _____ Transports urine from bladder to outside

K. _____ Region of the male urethra nearest the bladder

L. _____ Longest portion of the male urethra

Urine Formation

Match each of the three processes involved in urine formation with the correct description of that process.

1. _____ Solutes pass from tubular cells into the filtrate   A. glomerular filtration

2. _____ Solutes pass from the glomerulus into the capsule   B. tubular reabsorption

3. _____ Solutes pass from tubules into peritubular capillaries   C. tubular secretion

4. Write the terms that match the following phrases about the regulation of urine concentration and volume.

A. _____ Hormone that increases reabsorption of sodium

B. _____ Hormone that increases reabsorption of water

C. _____ Hormone that promotes sodium and water loss

D. _____ Enzyme produced by juxtaglomerular cells

E. _____ Powerful vasoconstrictor

F. _____ Act of expelling urine from the urinary bladder

5. Complete the following paragraph about tubular reabsorption and secretion by filling in the correct terms.

A. _____   E. _____

B. _____   F. _____

C. _____   G. _____

D. _____   H. _____

Tubular reabsorption moves substances from the filtrate into the blood and **A** the volume of urine. Water is reabsorbed by the process of **B**. Most of the solutes are reabsorbed by **C** mechanisms. Reabsorption of some solutes is limited by **D**. When concentration of these solutes exceeds **E**, the excess appears in the **F**. Tubular **G** adds substances to the urine. To help regulate blood pH, **H** ions are added to the urine and removed from the body by this process.

6. In what two ways does angiotensin II act on the kidneys?

A. _____

B. _____

Characteristics of Urine

1. Place a check (✓) before each of the following statements that is correct.

A. _____   The color of urine is due to urochrome.

B. _____   Urine is usually slightly acidic but may be alkaline.

C. _____   Normal urine volume is generally about 3 L per 24 hours.

D. _____   High-protein diets tend to make urine more alkaline.

E. _____   The specific gravity of urine is slightly greater than 1.

F. _____   Solutes make up about 20% of the urine volume.

G. _____   The predominant solute in urine is urea.

H. _____   In addition to urea, solutes in urine include glucose and albumin.

2. Write the clinical term that is used to indicate the presence of the following substances in the urine.

A. _____   White blood cells

B. _____   Albumin

C. _____   Glucose

D. _____   Erythrocytes

Body Fluids

1. List three types of sources for fluid intake. Place an asterisk (*) by the one that normally accounts for the greatest amount if intake.

   A. _____

   B. _____

   C. _____

2. List four avenues of fluid loss, and place an asterisk (*) by the one that normally accounts for the greatest amount of loss.

   A. _____

   B. _____

   C. _____

   D. _____

3. Write the terms that match the following phases about electrolytes in the body.

   A. _____   Predominant cation in extracellular fluid

   B. _____   Predominant anion in extracellular fluid

   C. _____   Predominant cation in intracellular fluid

   D. _____   Predominant anion in intracellular fluid

   E. _____   Primary hormone that regulates electrolytes

4. Write the terms that match the following phrases about acid-base balance in the body

   A. _____   Normal pH range of the blood

   B. _____   Clinical term for higher than normal pH

   C. _____   Clinical term for lower than normal pH

   D. _____   Primary regulators of blood pH (3)

   _____

   _____

5. Sarah has diabetes mellitus, which she finds difficult to control. On her last visit to her physician, she had ketosis and a below-normal blood pH. She also exhibited an increased respiratory rate.

   A. What is ketosis?

   _____

255

B. What acid-base imbalance does she have?

_____

C. Is this a respiratory or metabolic imbalance?

_____

D. Why is the respiratory rate increased?

_____

_____

6. Based on blood gas values alone, what is the preliminary diagnosis of the following? Indicate whether it is acidosis or alkalosis and whether it is respiratory or metabolic.

A. pH = 7.25 P_{CO_2} = 55.4 mm Hg HCO_3^- = 24.3 mEq/L   _____

B. pH = 7.26 P_{CO_2} = 40 mm Hg HCO_3^- = 7.1 mEq/L   _____

C. pH = 7.58 P_{CO_2} = 42 mm Hg HCO_3^- = 44 mEq/L   _____

D. pH = 7.56 P_{CO_2} = 23 mm Hg HCO_3^- = 23 mEq/L   _____

E. pH = 7.31 P_{CO_2} = 38 mm Hg HCO_3^- = 16 mEq/L   _____

7. Based on blood gas values and medical history, what is the preliminary diagnosis of the following? Indicate whether it is acidosis or alkalosis, respiratory or metabolic, and uncompensated or compensated.

A. A healthy 37-year-old man is having an elective open cholecystectomy under an anesthetic.

Blood gas values are pH = 7.10, P_{CO_2} = 70 mm Hg, and HCO_3^- = 27 mEq/L

_____

B. A 75-year-old man with a long history of chronic obstructive pulmonary disease is admitted to the hospital with fever and respiratory distress.

Blood gas values are pH = 7.10, P_{CO_2} = 75 mm Hg, and HCO_3^- = 30 mEq/L

_____

C. A 44-year-old moderately dehydrated man was admitted with a 2-day history of acute severe diarrhea.

Blood gas values were pH = 7.36, P_{CO_2} = 31 mm Hg, and HCO_3^- = 16 mEq/L

_____

D. An elderly woman from a nursing home was transferred to the hospital because of profound weakness and areflexia. Her oral intake had been poor for a few days.

Blood gas values were pH = 7.44, P_{CO_2} = 49 mm Hg, and HCO_3^- = 44.4 mEq/L

_____

E. A 19-year-old pregnant insulin-dependent diabetic patient was admitted with a history of polyuria and thirst. There is a history of poor compliance with medical therapy.

Blood gas values were pH = 7.26, P_{CO_2} = 16 mm Hg, and HCO_3^- = 7.1 mEq/L

_____

LABELING & COLORING EXERCISES

Identify the parts of the kidney by matching the letters from Figure 18-1 with the correct structure in the list.

1. _____ Major calyx

2. _____ Minor calyx

3. _____ Renal capsule

4. _____ Renal column

5. _____ Renal cortex

6. _____ Renal papilla

7. _____ Renal pelvis

8. _____ Renal pyramid

9. _____ Ureter

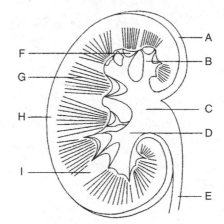

Figure 18-1 Coronal section through a kidney.

Identify the parts of a nephron by matching the letters from Figure 18-2 with the correct structure in the list. Draw a box around the renal corpuscle. Draw a circle around the region of the juxtaglomerular apparatus. Use blue to color the portions that are located in the medulla of the kidney.

10. _____ Afferent arteriole

11. _____ Ascending limb

12. _____ Collecting duct

13. _____ Descending limb

14. _____ Distal convoluted tubule

15. _____ Efferent arteriole

16. _____ Glomerular capsule

17. _____ Glomerulus

18. _____ Nephron loop

19. _____ Proximal convoluted tubule

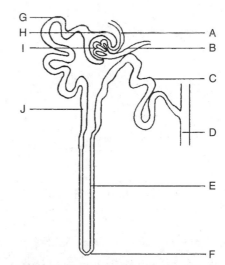

Figure 18-2 Diagram of a nephron.

20. Figure 18-3 illustrates a glomerulus with the glomerular capsule around it. Representative osmotic and hydrostatic pressures also are indicated. Draw red circles around the pressures that move substances from the glomerulus into the capsule, and draw blue circles around the pressures that move substances from the capsule into the glomerulus.

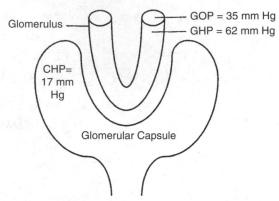

Glomerulus

GOP = 35 mm Hg
GHP = 62 mm Hg

CHP= 17 mm Hg

Glomerular Capsule

Figure 18-3 Representative pressures in glomerular filtration.

Calculate the net filtration pressure.
Net filtration pressure = _____

The boxes in Figure 18-4 represent the volume of different fluid compartments in the body. Match the letter of each box with the correct name. Also indicate the percent of total body weight that is contained in each compartment.

Compartment	Letter	Percent
21. Extracellular	_____	_____
22. Interstitial	_____	_____
23. Intracellular	_____	_____
24. Plasma	_____	_____
25. Solutes	_____	_____
26. Total fluids	_____	_____

A

B

C

D   E

F

Figure 18-4 Body fluid compartments.

27. Table 18-1 represents a nephron tubule and a blood capillary. Draw arrows to indicate whether substances move from the capillary into the tubule or from the tubule into the capillary in each of the three steps in urine formation.

	Glomerular Filtration	**Tubular Reabsorption**	**Tubular Secretion**
Capillary			
Tubule			

REVIEW QUESTIONS

1. What is the. principal function of the urinary system?

   _____

   _____

   _____

2. List the components of the urinary system in the sequence in which urine flows through them.

   _____   _____

   _____   _____

3. Describe the location of the kidneys relative to the peritoneum, thoracic vertebrae, and lumbar vertebrae.

   _____

   _____

   _____

4. Identify the regions of the kidney: cortex, medulla, renal column, renal pyramid, capsule, and the major and minor calyces.

   _____

5. What are the parts of a (a) renal corpuscle and (b) renal tubule?

   _____

   _____

6. Starting with the glomerular capsule, trace the flow of the filtrate through the kidney to the ureter.

   _____

   _____

7. What two regions are modified to form the juxtaglomerular apparatus? What does it secrete?

   _____

   _____

8. The afferent arterioles are branches of what vessels?

   _____

9. Where are the ureters located relative to the peritoneum? Where do they enter the urinary bladder?

   _____

   _____

10. Where is the detrusor muscle located?

   _____

259

11. What is the trigone?

_____

_____

12. What is the difference between the muscle in the internal urethral sphincter and the muscle in the external urethral sphincter?

_____

_____

13. What is micturition?

_____

_____

14. What are the three parts of the male urethra?

_____

_____

_____

15. What are the three processes that are involved in urine formation?

_____

_____

_____

16. How much glomerular filtrate is formed in a 24-hour period?

_____

17. What two components of blood normally are absent from the glomerular filtrate?

_____

18. What two pressures are inversely related to net filtration pressure? In other words, when the two pressures increase, the net filtration pressure decreases.

_____

_____

19. Where does *most* tubular reabsorption take place?

_____

20. What causes glucose to appear in the urine?

_____

_____

_____

21. By what transport mechanism is water reabsorbed?

_____

22. Where in the nephron tubule is water not reabsorbed?

_____

23. What process of urine formation adds substances to the filtrate?

_____

24. If blood volume or pressure decreases, what is likely to happen to urine volume? Explain.

_____

_____

_____

25. What three hormones act on the kidney tubules to regulate tubular reabsorption?

_____

_____

26. What is the purpose of renin?

_____

_____

27. What effect does angiotensin II have on the adrenal cortex?

_____

_____

28. How does solute concentration affect the specific gravity of the urine?

_____

_____

29. What terms describe the appearance of the following constituents in the urine: (a) red blood cells, (b) glucose, (c) albumin, (d) white blood cells?

_____

_____

_____

_____

30. Which fluid compartment has the most volume?

_____

31. In general, what accounts for the most fluid intake? Fluid loss?

_____

_____

32. What is the predominant (a) cation in extracellular fluid, (b) cation in intracellular fluid, (c) anion in extracellular fluid, (d) anion in intracellular fluid?

_____

_____

_____

_____

33. What term is used to designate a blood pH of 7.33?

_____

34. How does the urinary system respond if blood pH is too acidic?

_____

_____

35. Name four types of acid-base imbalance and the indicators for each type.

_____

_____

_____

_____

FUNCTIONAL RELATIONSHIPS

It is important to remember that no system in the body works alone. It takes the interaction of all systems to maintain homeostasis. The following exercises reinforce the concept that all systems work together to maintain the health and well-being of other systems and the individual.

Match the system on the right with what it provides for the urinary system on the left. Use the functional relationships page in your concepts textbook as a resource.

1. _____   Alternate excretory route for salts and nitrogenous wastes   A. Cardiovascular

2. _____   Supports and protects organs of the urinary system   B. Digestive

                                                                                  C. Endocrine
3. _____   Sphincters control voluntary urination
                                                                                  D. Integumentary
4. _____   Controls renal blood pressure; regulates bladder emptying   E. Lymphatic

                                                                                  F. Muscular
5. _____   Products regulate urine formation in the kidney
                                                                                  G. Nervous

6. _____ Delivers wastes to be excreted by the kidney

7. _____ Provides defense mechanisms against urinary tract pathogens

8. _____ Assists in regulating pH by removing carbon dioxide

9. _____ Metabolizes hormones, toxins, and drugs to forms that can be excreted in urine

10. _____ Portions surround the urethra in males

H. Reproductive
I. Respiratory
J. Skeletal

2. For each of the following systems, write what the urinary system provides for it.

A. Cardiovascular _____

B. Digestive _____

C. Reproductive _____

D. Endocrine _____

E. Lymphatic _____

F. Muscular _____

G. Nervous _____

H. Respiratory _____

I. Skeletal _____

J. Integumentary _____

REPRESENTATIVE DISORDERS

Match the disorder of the respiratory system on the right with its description of the left.

1. _____ Hereditary disease in which there is an enlargement of the kidney with the formation of cysts

2. _____ Inflammation of the urinary bladder

3. _____ Condition characterized by the presence of kidney stones

4. _____ Condition characterized by excessive protein in the urine

5. _____ Condition characterized by the deficiency of a hormone from the adrenal cortex

6. _____ Caused by a deficiency of antidiuretic hormone

7. _____ Inflammation of the urethra

8. _____ Inflammation of the capillary loops in the renal corpuscle

A. Cystitis
B. Diabetes insipidus
C. Glomerulonephritis
D. Hypoaldosteronism
E. Nephrolithiasis
F. Nephrotic syndrome
G. Polycystic kidney
H. Urethritis

Match the definitions on the left with the correct clinical term from the column on the right by placing the corresponding letter in the space before the definition. Not all terms will be used.

1. _____ Plasma

2. _____ Functional unit of the kidney

3. _____ Increased amounts of nitrogenous waste products in the blood

4. _____ Producing small amounts of urine

5. _____ Crushing of a calculus in kidney or bladder

6. _____ May be caused by hyperventilation

7. _____ Associated with defective uric acid metabolism

8. _____ Increases the production of urine

9. _____ Visual examination of the urinary bladder

10. _____ Involuntary emission of urine; bedwetting

A. Acidosis

B. Alkalosis

C. Azotemia

D. Cystoscopy

E. Diuretic

F. Enuresis

G. Glomerulus

H. Gout

I. Intracellular fluid

J. Intravascular fluid

K. Lithotripsy

L. Nephron

M. Oliguria

Write the meaning of the following abbreviations.

11. _____ BUN

12. _____ ARF

13. _____ GFR

14. _____ TUR

15. _____ UTI

16. _____ CRF

17. _____ IVP

18. _____ ADH

19. _____ ESRD

20. _____ UA

21. Spelling is important in scientific and medical applications because only one or two incorrect letters can change the meaning. Circle the correctly spelled word for each of the following pairs.

A. detrusor   detrussor

B. macula densa   macula denca

C. triagone   trigone

D. natriuretic   natrietic

E. albuminuria   albuminaria

22. Write the meaning of the underlined portion of each word on the line preceding the word.

A. _____ nephroptosis   F. _____ nocturia

B. _____ cystitis   G. _____ peritubular

C. _____ pyelolithotomy   H. _____ nephropexy

D. _____ nephrolithiasis I. _____ ureterorrhaphy

E. _____ azotemia   J. _____ juxtaglomeular

23. For each of the following words, underline the word part that corresponds to the underlined word or phrase in the definition.

    A. urethratresia   lack of an opening in the urethra

    B. chromaturia   abnormal color of the urine

    C. cystectasia   dilation of the urinary bladder

    D. micturition   to pass urine; urination

    E. oliguria   little urine, diminished urine production

    F. urethrophraxis   obstruction of the urethra

    G. nocturia   excessive urine at night

    H. cystopexy   surgical fixation of the bladder to the abdominal wall

    I. incontinence   inability to hold, or control, excretory functions

    J. azoturia   excessive nitrogen compounds (urea) in the urine

24. What is the clinical term for each of the following conditions or procedures?

    A. Rhea Knull experiences excessive urination during the night. _____

    B. Jose has inflammation of the capillary loops in the glomeruli of the kidney. _____

    C. Rocky has kidney stones. _____

    D. Polly has an enlarged kidney with numerous cysts. Her mother had the same condition and died of renal failure. _____

    E. Rena had a blood test to determine the effectiveness of her renal function. _____

    F. Allie has impaired kidney function and has to go to a center three times a week to have waste materials removed from the blood. _____

G. The physician suspected that Travis had an abnormality in the urinary system and ordered a radiographic procedure that uses a radiopaque dye injected into a vein so the renal vessels and urinary tract could be visualized. _____

H. Cal had kidney stones, so his physician ordered a procedure to crush the stones into small pieces that would be able to pass through the urinary tract and be excreted. _____

I. Betty had a metabolic condition characterized by polyuria and polydipsia. It was caused by a deficiency of a hormone secreted by the neurohypophysis. _____

J. Fran had to have her right kidney surgically removed. _____

TESTING COMPREHENSION

Multiple choice: Select the best response.

1. The functional unit of the kidney is the (a) pyramid, (b) collecting duct, (c) renal corpuscle, (d) nephron.

2. The renal sinus contains the (a) renal pelvis, (b) renal corpuscle, (c) renal pyramid, (d) renal papillae.

3. The portion of a nephron that is located in the medulla is the (a) glomerulus, (b) nephron loop of Henle, (c) proximal convoluted tubule, (d) distal convoluted tubule.

4. A renal corpuscle is composed of the (a) proximal and distal convoluted tubules, (b) collecting ducts, (c) glomerulus and glomerular capsule, (d) macula densa and juxtaglomerular cells.

5. The macula densa is located in the (a) afferent arteriole, (b) efferent arteriole, (c) ascending limb of the nephron loop, (d) descending limb of the nephron loop.

6. The arteries in the renal columns are the (a) interlobar arteries, (b) segmental arteries, (c) interlobular arteries, (d) arcuate arteries.

7. Renin is produced by specialized cells in the (a) medulla, (b) nephron loop, (c) macula densa, (d) afferent arteriole.

8. A hormone produced by the kidneys is (a) renin, (b) erythropoietin, (c) angiotensin, (d) aldosterone.

9. The smooth muscle in the wall of the urinary bladder is the (a) detrusor, (b) sphincter, (c) trigone, (d) rugae.

10. The voluntary sphincter of the urethra is (a) the internal sphincter, (b) the external sphincter, (c) composed of smooth muscle, (d) detrusor muscle.

11. The proximal, or first, portion of the male urethra is the (a) prostatic urethra, (b) penile urethra, (c) spongy urethra, (d) membranous urethra.

12. If the glomerular osmotic pressure is 35 mm Hg, glomerular hydrostatic pressure is 62 mm Hg, and the capsular hydrostatic pressure is 17 mm Hg, then the net filtration pressure is (a) 52 mm Hg, (b) 97 mm Hg, (c) 10 mm Hg, (d) 18 mm Hg.

13. Urine volume will be increased if there is (a) increased tubular reabsorption of water, (b) increased secretion of renin, (c) increased secretion of antidiuretic hormone, (d) increased glomerular hydrostatic pressure.

14. The hormone that promotes sodium and water loss in the urine is (a) aldosterone, (b) antidiuretic hormone, (c) atrial natriuretic hormone, (d) angiotensin.

15. The predominate solute in urine is (a) urea, (b) albumin, (c) urochrome, (d) glucose.

16. The presence of leukocytes in the urine is called (a) albuminuria, (b) pyuria, (c) oliguria, (d) hematuria.

17. For a normal adult male who weighs 80 kg (176 lb), the volume of fluid in his body is about (a) 48 L, (b) 32 L, (c) 16 L, (d) 60 L.

18. For a normal adult man who weighs 80 kg (176 lb), the volume of extracellular fluid is about (a) 48 L; (b) 32 L; (c) 16 L, (d) 5 L.

19. The thirst center for regulation of fluid intake is located in the (a) parotid gland, (b) aortic bodies, (c) pons, (d) hypothalamus.

20. The primary cation in extracellular fluid is (a) sodium, (b) potassium, (c) phosphate, (d) bicarbonate.

21. The primary anion in intracellular fluid is (a) sodium, (b) potassium, (c) phosphate, (d) bicarbonate.

22. Aldosterone influences urine volume by (a) increasing the reabsorption of sodium, (b) decreasing glomerular filtration rate, (c) increasing reabsorption of water in the ascending limb of the nephron loop, (d) increasing the secretion of antidiuretic hormone.

23. The normal pH of blood is (a) 7.0, (b) 7.2, (c) 7.4, (d) 7.6.

24. Blood gas values of pH = 7.6, P_{CO_2} = 40 mm Hg, and HCO_3^- = 28 mEq/L indicate (a) respiratory acidosis, (b) respiratory alkalosis, (c) metabolic acidosis, (d) metabolic alkalosis.

25. Hysterical hyperventilation may lead to (a) respiratory acidosis, (b) respiratory alkalosis, (c) metabolic acidosis, (d) metabolic alkalosis.

A STEP BEYOND

Go a step beyond the ordinary and learn more about a topic that is related to this chapter but not discussed in detail in the textbook. Select one of the following topics, or one suggested by your instructor, and write a brief paper (250 words minimum), create a poster, or develop a short presentation (approximately 4 to 5 minutes) that focuses on your selection. Suggested topics for this chapter:

1. *Kangaroo rats*. Kangaroo rats are unique in the animal world because they have the ability to survive with little or no water. They do not store water in their bodies, yet their bodies have about the same water content as other animals. What are Kangaroo rats, and where do they live? How do they survive without water?
2. *Renal failure and anemia*. Chronic renal failure is usually accompanied by anemia. Why? How can the anemia be treated?
3. *Drug abuse*. How does drug abuse affect your kidneys? What drugs are harmful to your kidneys?
4. *Kidney transplants*. What is the history of kidney transplants? Answer the usual history questions of who, when, where, and the results. What are some of the ethical issues involved in kidney transplants?
5. *Dialysis*. What is dialysis? When was the first successful dialysis procedure performed? When is dialysis indicated? What is the difference between hemodialysis and peritoneal dialysis? How does each type work?

FUN & GAMES

Word Scramble

Determine the word that fits each definition, and then write the word in the spaces below the definition, one letter per space. The letters in the boxes form a scrambled word or words. Unscramble the letters to create a word (or words) that matches the final definition in each section.

1. Reduced urine output

2. Indentation on medial side of kidney

3. Hormone produced by the kidney

4. Arterioles that are branches of interlobular arteries

5. Inner region of the kidney

Letters to use for final words: _____

Final definition: First process in urine formation

_____

6. Primary organs of the urinary system

7. Outer region of the kidney

8. Cluster of capillaries in the renal corpuscle

9. Vessel that passes over the base of a renal pyramid

10. Circular bands of muscle that surround each end of the urethra

Letters to use for final words: _____

Final definition: Imbalance caused by hyperventilation

_____

19 Reproductive System

LEARNING EXERCISES

Overview of the Reproductive System

1. List four functions of the reproductive system.

   A. _____

   B. _____

   C. _____

   D. _____

2. What is the primary reproductive organ in the (A) male and (B) female?

   A. _____

   B. _____

Male Reproductive System

1. Number the following structures in the correct sequence, from 1 to 10, to trace the pathway of sperm from the seminiferous tubule to the exterior. Start with 1 for the seminiferous tubule.

   A. _____ Ductus deferens   F. _____ Penile urethra

   B. _____ Efferent ducts   G. _____ Prostatic urethra

   C. _____ Ejaculatory duct   H. _____ Rete testis

   D. _____ Epididymis   I. _____ Seminiferous tubules

   E. _____ Membranous urethra   J. _____ Straight tubules

2. Write the terms that match the following phrases about the male reproductive system.

   A. _____ Male gonad

   B. _____ Male gamete

   C. _____ Pouch of skin that contains the male gonad

   D. _____ Smooth muscle in subcutaneous tissue of scrotum

   E. _____ Skeletal muscle fibers in the spermatic cord

   F. _____ Fibrous connective tissue capsule of the testes

   G. _____ Specific location of spermatogenesis

269

H. _____ Cells that produce male sex hormones

I. _____ Maturation of spermatids into spermatozoa

J. _____ Region of spermatozoa that contains mitochondria

K. _____ Number of chromosomes in a spermatid

L. _____ Cells that nourish developing spermatids

3. Match each of the following phrases with the accessory gland to which it pertains.

A. _____ Product secreted into the penile urethra

B. _____ Encircles the proximal portion of the urethra

C. _____ Located posterior to the urinary bladder

D. _____ Secretion accounts for 60% of the seminal fluid

E. _____ Located near the base of the penis

F. _____ Smallest of the accessory glands

G. _____ Secretion has a high fructose content

1. seminal vesicles
2. prostate
3. bulbourethral gland

4. Complete the following paragraph about the male sexual response by filling in the correct terms.

During sexual stimulation $\underline{A}$ impulses dilate the $\underline{B}$ and constrict the $\underline{C}$ of the penis. This causes the spaces in the erectile tissue to fill with blood, and the penis enlarges and becomes rigid. This is called $\underline{D}$. With continued stimulation, these reflexes become more intense until they prompt a surge of $\underline{E}$ impulses to the genital organs. These impulses cause the forceful discharge of semen into the urethra. This is called $\underline{F}$. $\underline{G}$, the forceful expulsion of semen to the exterior, and it immediately follows. The muscular contractions that result in the expulsion of semen are accompanied by feelings of pleasure, $\underline{H}$ heart rate, $\underline{I}$ blood pressure, and $\underline{J}$. Collectively, these physiologic responses are referred to as $\underline{K}$.

A. _____   G. _____

B. _____   H. _____

C. _____   I. _____

D. _____   J. _____

E. _____   K. _____

F. _____

5. Write the terms that match the following phrases about the hormones that control male reproductive functions.

A. _____ Hypothalamic hormone that initiates puberty

B. _____ Hormone from the interstitial cells

C. _____ Hormone that stimulates the interstitial cells

270

Chapter **19** **Reproductive System**

D. _____ Collective term for male sex hormones

E. _____ With testosterone it stimulates spermatogenesis

F. _____ Anterior pituitary hormones that act on testes (2)

_____

G. _____ Source of testosterone before birth

H. _____ Functions of testosterone (2)

_____

Female Reproductive System

1. Write the terms that match the following phrases about the internal female reproductive system.

A. _____ Female gonad

B. _____ Stage of oogenesis present at birth

C. _____ Stage of oogenesis that is ovulated each month

D. _____ Clear glycoprotein membrane around an oocyte

E. _____ Cells around oocyte at ovulation

F. _____ Develops from follicle after ovulation

G. _____ Fingerlike extensions of the uterine tubes

H. _____ Opening from the cervix into the vagina

I. _____ Largest ligament that stabilizes the uterus

J. _____ Muscular layer of the uterus

K. _____ Endometrial region shed during menstruation

L. _____ Mucous membrane covering vaginal orifice

2. Write the terms that match the following phrases about the female external genitalia.

A. _____ Collective term for female external genitalia

B. _____ Fat-filled folds of skin that enclose the genitalia

C. _____ Mound of fat the overlies the symphysis pubis

D. _____ Area between the two labia minora

E. _____ Female structure homologous to male penis

F. _____ Glands adjacent to the urethral orifice

G. _____ Glands adjacent to the vaginal orifice

3. Write T before the true statements and F before the false statements about the female sexual response.

    A. _____ The female sexual response consists of erection and orgasm.

    B. _____ Sympathetic responses to sexual stimuli produce increased blood flow to erectile tissue.

    C. _____ Sympathetic responses produce rhythmic contractions of the uterus and pelvic floor, accompanied by feelings of intense pleasure.

4. Match the following statements and phrases with the correct hormone. Some may have more than one correct response. Give all correct answers.

    A. _____ Starts the events of puberty

    B. _____ Levels increase after menopause

    C. _____ Secreted by the hypothalamus

    D. _____ Secreted by the anterior pituitary

    E. _____ Triggers ovulation

    F. _____ Secreted by the corpus luteum

    G. _____ Secreted by cells of the ovarian follicle

    H. _____ Stimulates secretory phase of uterine cycle

    I. _____ Stimulates proliferative phase of uterine cycle

    J. _____ Stimulates development of the corpus luteum

    K. _____ Stimulates development of glandular tissue in the breast

    L. _____ Stimulates development of the duct system in the breast

    M. _____ Causes an accumulation of adipose tissue in the breast

    N. _____ Stimulates growth of ovarian follicles

    O. _____ Levels decrease after menopause

1. gonadotropin-releasing hormone
2. follicle-stimulating hormone
3. luteinizing hormone
4. estrogen
5. progesterone

5. Complete the following statements by using the words *increases* or *decreases*.

    A. As ovarian follicles grow in response to FSH, estrogen secretion _____.

    B. Blood estrogen level _____ during days 6 to 13 of the menstrual cycle.

    C. After ovulation, progesterone secretion _____.

    D. An increasing level of progesterone _____ LH secretion.

    E. The menstrual phase of the uterine cycle is caused by _____ in progesterone levels.

6. Write the terms that match the following phrases about the breast.

A. _____ Circular pigmented area around the nipple

B. _____ Bands of connective tissue that support the breast

C. _____ Collects the milk from the glandular units

D. _____ Dilated region of duct that is a reservoir for milk

E. _____ Hormone that stimulates milk production

F. _____ Hormone that causes ejection of milk from glands

LABELING & COLORING EXERCISES

Identify the parts of the male reproductive system by matching the letters from Figure 19-1 with the correct structure in the list.

1. _____ Bulbourethral gland

2. _____ Corpus cavernosum

3. _____ Corpus spongiosum

4. _____ Ductus deferens

5. _____ Ejaculatory duct

6. _____ Epididymis

7. _____ Glans penis

8. _____ Prostate

9. _____ Scrotum

10. _____ Symphysis pubis

11. _____ Testicle

12. _____ Urethra (2 places)

   _____

13. _____ Urinary bladder

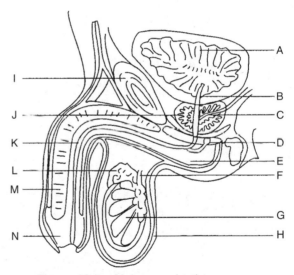

Figure 19-1 Male reproductive organs.

Chapter **19 Reproductive System**

Identify the parts of the female reproductive system by matching the letters from Figure 19-2 with the correct structure in the list.

14. _____ Cervix

15. _____ Clitoris

16. _____ Infundibulum

17. _____ Mons pubis

18. _____ Ovary

19. _____ Rectum

20. _____ Symphysis pubis

21. _____ Urethra

22. _____ Urinary bladder

23. _____ Uterine tube

24. _____ Uterus

25. _____ Vagina

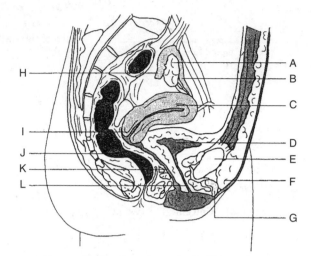

Figure 19-2 Female reproductive organs.

Identify the structures associated with the ovary and uterine tube by matching the letters from Figure 19-3 with the correct item in the list.

26. _____ Antrum

27. _____ Corpus albicans

28. _____ Corpus luteum

29. _____ Fimbriae

30. _____ Infundibulum

31. _____ Primary follicle

32. _____ Secondary follicle

33. _____ Secondary oocyte

34. _____ Uterine tube

35. _____ Vesicular follicle

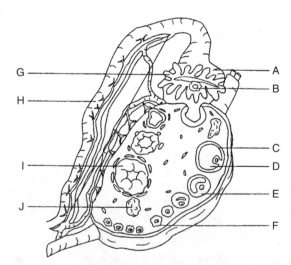

Figure 19-3 Ovary and uterine tube.

36. Figure 19-4 represents a sagittal section of the female breast. Color the adipose tissue yellow and the pectoralis major muscle red. Identify other structures as indicated.

A. _____

B. _____

C. _____

D. _____

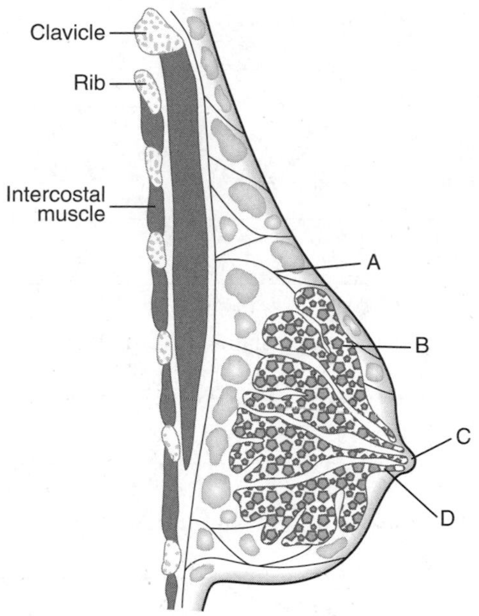

Clavicle

Rib

Intercostal muscle

A

B

C

D

Figure 19-4   Sagittal section of the female breast.

REVIEW QUESTIONS

1. What organs are the primary reproductive organs, and what is their function?

   _____

   _____

   _____

2. Identify the parts of the male reproductive system: testis, scrotum, epididymis, ductus deferens, prostate, prostatic urethra, ejaculatory duct, membranous urethra, bulbourethral gland, spongy urethra, and penis.

   _____

3. Where are the male gonads located early in their development? Where are they normally located at birth?

   _____

   _____

4. Where are the seminiferous tubules located, and what is their function?

   _____

   _____

5. How many chromosomes are in a (a) spermatogonium, (b) primary spermatocyte, (c) secondary spermatocyte, (d) spermatid, (e) spermatozoa?

   _____   _____

   _____   _____

   _____

6. In mature spermatozoa, what is contained in the (a) acrosome, (b) head, (c) midpiece?

_____

_____

_____

7. What duct do the sperm enter when they leave the (a) epididymis, (b) ejaculatory duct?

_____

_____

8. Which accessory gland makes the largest contribution to the seminal fluid? Where are these glands located?

_____

_____

9. In reference to seminal fluid, what is meant by the term *emission*?

_____

_____

10. What erectile tissue surrounds the urethra in the penis?

_____

11. What effects do FSH and LH have on the testes?

_____

_____

_____

12. Identify the parts of the female reproductive system: ovary, uterus, uterine tubes, mons pubis, cervix, vagina, urethra, labia majora, labia minora, clitoris, and mons pubis.

_____

13. What type of follicles is in the ovarian cortex of a normal 5-year-old girl?

_____

14. How many secondary oocytes are produced from each primary oocyte? How does this compare with the number of secondary spermatocytes that are produced from each primary spermatocyte?

_____

_____

_____

15. What two structures (or layers) surround the secondary oocyte in a vesicular follicle?

_____

16. At what stage of meiosis is the oocyte that is released at the time of ovulation?

_____

17. What portion of the uterine tubes is closest to the ovaries?

_____

18. What portion of the uterus is between the internal os and the external os?

_____

19. What specific portion of the uterine wall is sloughed off during menstruation?

_____

20. What are the purposes of the vagina? Where does it open to the exterior?

_____

_____

_____

21. What hormone is increasing during the follicular phase of the ovarian cycle?

_____

22. What phase of the uterine cycle corresponds to the luteal phase of the ovarian cycle? What hormones are increasing during this period?

_____

_____

23. What effects do estrogen and progesterone have on the structure of the mammary glands?

_____

_____

24. How does the posterior pituitary affect the mammary glands?

_____

_____

FUNCTIONAL RELATIONSHIPS

It is important to remember that no system in the body works alone. It takes the interaction of all systems to maintain homeostasis. The following exercises reinforce the concept that all systems work together to maintain the health and wellbeing of other systems and the individual.

Match the system on the right with what it provides for the reproductive system on the left. Use the functional relationships page in your concepts textbook as a resource.

1. _____ Transports reproductive hormones to target tissues

2. _____ Contractions contribute to orgasm in both sexes

3. _____ Protects testes, provides tactile sensations

4. _____ Maintains pH and electrolyte balance for gonadal hormone function

5. _____ Protection for pelvic reproductive organs

6. _____ Regulates sex drive, arousal, orgasm

7. _____ Defense against pathogens that enter through reproductive tract

8. _____ Major role in differentiation and development of reproductive organs

9. _____ Supplies oxygen for metabolism in reproductive organs

10. _____ Provides nutrients for growth and maintenance of reproductive tissues

A. Cardiovascular
B. Digestive
C. Endocrine
D. Integumentary
E. Lymphatic
F. Muscular
G. Nervous
H. Respiratory
I. Skeletal
J. Urinary

11. For each of the following systems, write what the reproductive system provides for it.

A. Cardiovascular _____

B. Digestive _____

C. Endocrine _____

D. Integumentary _____

E. Lymphatic _____

F. Muscular _____

G. Nervous _____

H. Respiratory _____

I. Skeletal _____

J. Urinary _____

REPRESENTATIVE DISORDERS

Match the disorder of the respiratory system on the right with its description of the left.

1. _____ Sexually transmitted disease (STD) caused by *Treponema pallidum*

2. _____ Tumors usually arise from germ cells in the male

3. _____ Tissue of uterine lining occurs in abnormal sites

4. _____ Excessive development of mammary glands in the male

5. _____ May be detected by dysplasia of epithelial cells in a Pap smear

6. _____ Testes fail to descend into the scrotum

7. _____ Malignancy arising from milk glands and ducts

8. _____ Symptoms result from increased gonadocorticoids

9. _____ Absence of menstruation

10. _____ Highly contagious and most prevalent STD in the United States

A. Adrenogenital syndrome

B. Amenorrhea

C. Breast cancer

D. Cryptorchidism

E. Endometriosis

F. Gonorrhea

G. Gynecomastia

H. Syphilis

I. Testicular cancer

J. Uterine cancer

VOCABULARY PRACTICE

Match the definitions on the left with the correct clinical term from the column on the right by placing the corresponding letter in the space before the definition. Not all terms will be used.

1. _____ Sex cells; sperm and ova

2. _____ Combination estrogen and progestin oral contraceptive that most closely resembles hormone levels during a normal monthly cycle

3. _____ Abdominal pain that may occur at time of ovulation

4. _____ Surgical removal of a testis

5. _____ Low sperm count

6. _____ Primary reproductive organs

7. _____ Synthetic progesterone

8. _____ Surgical removal of a uterine tube

9. _____ Removal of a growth or other matter from the uterus by scraping or suction

10. _____ Sexual intercourse between a man and a woman

A. Coitus

B. Curettage

C. Gametes

D. Gonads

E. Mittelschmerz

F. Monophasic

G. Oligospermia

H. Orchiectomy

I. Phimosis

J. Progestin

K. Salpingectomy

L. Triphasic

11. Write the meaning of the following abbreviations.

A. _____ PMS

B. _____ STD

C. _____ VD

D. _____ IUD

E. _____ PID

F. _____ D&C

G. _____ IVF

H. _____ PSA

I. _____ BSE

J. _____ TAH

12. Spelling is important in scientific and medical applications because only one or two incorrect letters can change the meaning. Circle the correctly spelled word for each of the following pairs.

A. menarche   menarch   F. semineferous   seminiferous

B. primodial   primordial   G. epididymis   epidydimis

C. pudenum   pudendum   H. mammry   mammary

D. hysterectomy   histerectomy   I. antiflexed   anteflexed

E. prostate   prostrate   J. perimetrium   parametrium

13. Write the meaning of the underlined portion of each word on the line preceding the word.

A. _____ <u>men</u>opause

B. _____ <u>fimbri</u>ae

C. _____ <u>colp</u>oscopy

D. _____ <u>lapar</u>oscopy

E. _____ <u>epis</u>iotomy

F. _____ crypt<u>orchid</u>ism

G. _____ <u>crypt</u>orchidism

H. _____ <u>balan</u>itis

I. _____ hypo<u>spadias</u>

J. _____ <u>ejacul</u>ation

14. For each of the following words, underline the word part that corresponds to the underlined word or phrase in the definition.

A. hysterectomy   surgical removal of the <u>uterus</u>

B. oophorectomy   surgical removal of an <u>ovary</u>

C. salpingolithiasis   presence of calcium deposits in the uterine <u>tube</u>

280

D. myometrium	muscle layer of the <u>uterine</u> wall
E. androgens	hormones that produce <u>male</u> characteristics
F. balanitis	inflammation of the <u>glans</u> penis
G. gynecogenic	producing <u>female</u> characteristics
H. orchiopathy	any disease of the <u>testes</u>
I. hypospadias	urethral <u>opening</u> is on the undersurface of the penis
J. mammogram	a radiograph of the <u>breast</u>

Answer the following questions.

15. James had an enlarged prostate gland, and his physician ordered a blood test for prostate specific antigen (PSA). It was determined that he had benign prostatic hypertrophy and treatment included a transurethral prostatectomy (TURP).

    A. What is PSA?

    _____

    _____

    B. What is TURP?

    _____

    _____

16. Carol, who is 23, is athletic and trains regularly for running marathons. Now she is concerned because it has been 3 months since her last menstrual period and she is not pregnant.
    What is the clinical term for her condition?

    _____

TESTING COMPREHENSION

Multiple choice: Select the best response.

1. The primary reproductive organ in the male is the (a) penis, (b) testicle, (c) ductus deferens, (d) spermatozoon.

2. Testes begin their development in the (a) abdomen, near the kidney; (b) pelvic cavity near the urinary bladder; (c) scrotum, near the epididymis; (d) pelvic cavity, near the prostate.

3. The smooth muscle in the wall of the scrotum is the (a) detrusor muscle, (b) cremaster muscle, (c) dartos muscle, (d) rectus abdominis muscle.

4. Which of the following best describes a difference between spermatogenesis and oogenesis? (a) the primary spermatocyte produces four spermatids but a primary oocyte produces only two ova; (b) all primary spermatocytes develop after puberty but all primary oocytes develop before birth; (c) secondary spermatocytes have 46 chromosomes, but secondary oocytes have only 23; (d) LH stimulates spermatogenesis but FSH stimulates oogenesis.

5. Arrange the given ducts in the correct sequence for the passage of sperm: (1) ejaculatory duct, (2) epididymis, (3) urethra, (4) ductus deferens, (5) efferent duct. (a) 2, 4, 1, 3, 5; (b) 4, 5, 2, 1, 3; (c) 5, 2, 4, 3, 1; (d) 5, 2, 4, 1, 3.

6. The prostate gland (a) empties into the penile urethra, (b) contributes about 60% of the volume of seminal fluid, (c) secretes a thin, milky-colored fluid, (d) is located posterior to the urinary bladder.

7. Seminal vesicles (a) encircle the urethra, (b) empty into the spongy urethra, (c) contribute the smallest volume of seminal fluid, (d) secrete a viscous fluid that contains fructose.

8. Mitochondria that produce adenosine triphosphate for sperm are located in the (a) midpiece, (b) acrosome, (c) head, (d) tail.

9. In the penis, corpus spongiosum (a) forms two ventral columns, (b) forms a single dorsal column, (c) makes up the glans penis, (d) has no vascular sinusoids.

10. Emission and ejaculation are accomplished by (a) sympathetic nerve impulses to the ducts and accessory glands, (b) sympathetic nerve impulses dilating the arterioles that supply blood to the penis, (c) parasympathetic nerve impulses that constrict the veins in the penis, (d) parasympathetic nerve impulses to the skeletal muscle in the wall of the urethra.

11. In the male, FSH (a) stimulates the production of testosterone, (b) stimulates spermatogenesis, (c) promotes male secondary sex characteristics, (d) promotes glandular secretion of the interstitial cells.

12. In men, LH (a) stimulates secretion of FSH, (b) promotes development of male secondary sex characteristics, (c) stimulates the interstitial cells, (d) promotes development of sustentacular cells.

13. The female gonad is the (a) ovary, (b) uterus, (c) pudendum, (d) vagina.

14. At birth the ovaries contain (a) oogonia, (b) primary oocytes, (c) secondary oocytes, (d) primary follicles.

15. The noncellular layer that surrounds the oocyte at the time of ovulation is the (a) corona radiata, (b) zona pellucida, (c) granulosa, (d) antrum.

16. The infundibulum is a part of the (a) ovary, (b) uterus, (c) vagina, (d) uterine tube.

17. The muscular wall of the uterus is the (a) endometrium, (b) stratum functionale, (c) stratum basale, (d) myometrium.

18. The largest ligament that holds the uterus in place is the (a) broad ligament, (b) suspensory ligament, (c) round ligament, (d) cardinal ligament.

19. The portion of the uterus between the internal os and the external os is the (a) vagina, (b) cervix, (c) fundus, (d) body.

20. The portion of the uterine wall that changes during the uterine cycle is the (a) perimetrium, (b) stratum basale, (c) stratum functionale, (d) myometrium.

21. Which of the following is *not* correct about the vulva? (a) the opening for the vagina is anterior to the urethra, (b) labia majora have an abundance of adipose, (c) labia minora form a prepuce over the clitoris, (d) the clitoris is the most anterior structure in the vestibule.

22. Ovulation occurs as a result of (a) declining levels of estrogen, (b) high levels of progesterone, (c) a rapid increase in LH, (d) low levels of FSH.

23. The luteal phase of the ovarian cycle corresponds to the (a) menstrual phase of the uterine cycle, (b) proliferative phase of the uterine cycle, (c) the secretory phase of the uterine cycle, (d) the follicular phase of the uterine cycle.

24. During the proliferative phase of the uterine cycle, (a) menstruation occurs, (b) estrogen levels increase, (c) the corpus luteum develops, (d) the corpus luteum secretes progesterone.

25. The development of glandular tissue in the female breast is stimulated by (a) prolactin, (b) luteinizing hormone, (c) progesterone, (d) estrogen.

Go a step beyond the ordinary and learn more about a topic that is related to this chapter but not discussed in detail in the textbook. Select one of the following topics, or one suggested by your instructor, and write a brief paper (250 words minimum), create a poster, or develop a short presentation (approximately 4-5 minutes) that focuses on your selection. Suggested topics for this chapter:

1. Endometriosis. What is it? What is the cause? Can it be cured? How can it be treated? Investigate endometriosis and discover the answers to these questions.
2. Oligospermia. What is it? How common is it? What are some of the causes? How can it be treated?
3. Syphilis. What is the etiology of this STD? Describe the three stages in the pathogenesis of syphilis.
4. Syphilis. Many notable people from history either died of syphilis or were suspected to have had syphilis. Select one of these and do a biographical sketch focusing on the impact that syphilis had on their lives. Suggestions include, but are not limited to, Napoleon Bonaparte, Al Capone, Paul Gaugin, Adolph Hitler, Scott Joplin, Edouard Manet, Jack Pickford, and Franz Schubert.
5. STDs. Select three STDs other than syphilis and investigate the etiology, signs, symptoms, pathogenesis, and treatment of each one.

FUN & GAMES

Word Scramble

Determine the word that fits each definition, and then write the word in the spaces across from the definition, one letter per space. The letters in the boxes form a scrambled word or words. Unscramble the letters to create a word (or words) that matches the final definition in each section.

1. Egg and sperm cells

2. Male accessory gland that surrounds the urethra

3. Muscle in the spermatic cord

4. Congenital absence of the testes

5. Location of the testes

Letters to use for final word: _____

Final definition: Meiosis in the male

_____

6. Clear membrane around the oocyte

7. Connective tissue capsule around the ovary

8. Inner region of an ovary

9. Homologous to the male penis

10. Type of tissue in the endometrium

Letters to use for final word: _____

Final definition: Abdominal pain at ovulation

_____

20 Development and Heredity

LEARNING EXERCISES

Fertilization

1. Write the terms that match the following phrases about fertilization.

A. _____   Single cell that is product of fertilization

B. _____   Cells that surround ovulated secondary oocyte

C. _____   Process that weakens acrosomal membrane

D. _____   Length of time ovulated oocytes are fertile

E. _____   Usual site of fertilization

Pre-Embryonic Period

1. Write the terms that match the following phrases about the pre-embryonic period.

A. _____   Developments during pre-embryonic period (3)

   _____

   _____

B. _____   Early cell divisions of the zygote

C. _____   Cells that are the result of cleavage

D. _____   Solid ball of cells resulting from cell division

E. _____   Hollow sphere of cells formed by fifth day

F. _____   Cluster of cells that becomes embryo

G. _____   Cavity within hollow sphere of cells

H. _____   Flattened cells around cavity of blastocyst

I. _____   Blastocyst cells that contribute to placenta

J. _____   Layer of uterine wall where implantation occurs

K. _____   Hormone secreted by the blastocyst

L. _____   Hormone that maintains the uterine lining

M. _____ Cluster of cells that forms primary germ layers

N. _____ Primary germ layers (3)

_____

_____

Embryonic Development

1. Complete the following statements by writing the correct words in the blanks.

The period of embryonic development lasts from the beginning of the _____ week after conception

to the end of the _____ week. Three significant developments during this period are the formation

of the _____ membranes, formation of the _____, and formation of all the body

_____ systems. During this period the developing offspring is called a/an _____.

2. Match each of the following descriptive phrases with the correct extraembryonic membrane from the list.

A. _____ Forms a sac around the developing embryo   1. amnion

B. _____ Produces the primordial germ cells   2. allantois

C. _____ Becomes part of the umbilical cord   3. chorion

D. _____ Develops from the trophoblast   4. yolk sac

E. _____ Cushions and protects developing offspring

F. _____ Contributes to the formation of the placenta

G. _____ Develops fingerlike projections called villi

H. _____ Filled with fluid

3. Complete the following paragraph about the placenta by filling in the correct terms.

The placenta develops as <u>A</u> from the embryo penetrate the <u>B</u> of the uterus. The <u>C</u> become highly vascular and extend to the <u>D</u> arteries and veins. The spaces in the endometrium are filled with maternal <u>E</u>. This interface allows <u>F</u> and nutrients to diffuse from the mother's blood into the fetal blood. Metabolic wastes and <u>G</u> diffuse from the <u>H</u> into the <u>I</u>.

A. _____   F. _____

B. _____   G. _____

C. _____   H. _____

D. _____   I. _____

E. _____

4. Match each of the following tissues with the primary germ layer from which it is derived.

A. _____ Epithelial lining of the digestive tract   1. ectoderm

B. _____ Epidermis of the skin   2. mesoderm

C. _____ Cardiac muscle   3. endoderm

D. _____ Nervous tissue

E. _____ Cartilage

F. _____ Hair, nails, glands of the skin

G. _____ Respiratory epithelium

H. _____ Epithelium lining the blood vessels

I. _____ Lining of the oral cavity

J. _____ Bone

K. _____ Dermis of the skin

L. _____ Epithelial lining of the vagina

Fetal Development

1. Write the terms that match the following phrases about fetal development.

A. _____ First recognizable movements of fetus

B. _____ Protective coating over fetal skin

C. _____ Opening between the atria in the fetus

D. _____ Transports blood from placenta to fetus

E. _____ Allows blood to bypass fetal liver

Parturition and Lactation

1. Write the terms that match the following phrases about labor and delivery.

A. _____ Process of giving birth to an infant

B. _____ Series of contractions to expel fetus

C. _____ Hormone that inhibits uterine contractions

D. _____ Sensitizes uterus to effects of oxytocin

E. _____ Secretes oxytocin

F. _____ Act with oxytocin to stimulate contractions

G. _____ Type of feedback between oxytocin and uterus

H. _____ Longest stage of labor

I. _____ Stage of labor in which fetus is delivered

J. _____ Stage characterized by rhythmic contractions

K. _____ Final stage of labor

L. _____ Normal position, or presentation, of baby

2. Complete the following paragraph about the changes that take place in the lungs immediately after birth.

The fetal lungs are A and nonfunctional. When the B is cut, the oxygen supply from the mother ceases. Increasing C levels, decreasing D, and E oxygen stimulate the respiratory center in the F. The respiratory muscles contract and the baby takes its first breath. Usually this is strong and deep and inflates the alveoli.

A. _____   D. _____

B. _____   E. _____

C. _____   F. _____

3. Write the terms that match the following phrases about lactation.

A. _____   Refers to the production and ejection of milk

B. _____   Hormone that stimulates milk production

C. _____   Hormone that stimulates milk ejection

D. _____   Inhibit milk production during pregnancy (2)

   _____

E. _____   Yellowish fluid secreted before milk begins

4. Complete the following paragraph about the stimulation for milk production.

Each time a mother nurses her infant, impulses from the nipple to the <u>A</u> stimulate the release of <u>B</u>. This causes a temporary increase in <u>C</u>, which stimulates <u>D</u> for the next nursing period. If a mother stops nursing her baby, milk production <u>E</u> within a few <u>F</u>.

A. _____   D. _____

B. _____   E. _____

C. _____   F. _____

Postnatal Development

1. Identify the period of postnatal development described by each of the following.

A. _____   Lasts for about a month after birth

B. _____   Period of old age

C. _____   Lasts from the end of first year until puberty

D. _____   Lasts from the end of first month to end of first year

E. _____ Puberty until adulthood

F. _____ Body weight generally triples

G. _____ Bladder and bowel controls are established

H. _____ Degenerative changes become significant

Heredity

Match each of the following terms with its definition.

1. _____ Two or more alternative forms of genes   A. alleles

2. _____ Entire collection of genetic material in a cell   B. autosomes

3. _____ Twenty-two pairs of chromosomes in humans   C. genome

4. _____ X and Y chromosomes   D. hereditary disorder

5. _____ Two alleles of a pair are identical   E. homozygous

6. _____ Expression of genes   F. mutation

7. _____ Traits that are governed by more than one pair of genes   G. phenotype

8. _____ Traits are carried on X and Y chromosomes   H. polygenic

9. _____ A change in an individual's genetic code   I. sex chromosomes

10. _____ Cystic fibrosis, hemophilia, and phenylketonuria   J. sex-linked inheritance

11. Use Punnett squares to answer the following questions:

A. Assume that eye color is a monogenic autosomal trait and that brown is dominant over blue. Two parents are heterozygous for brown eyes. What proportion of their children will have brown eyes and what portion will have blue eyes?

_____

_____

B. Shari has type AB blood. Her fiancé is also type AB. What are the possible blood types for their children?

_____

_____

C. Jace and his mother have normal color vision. His brother and sister are color blind. What are the genotypes of Jace's mother, father, brother, and sister? Assume that color blindness is an X-linked recessive trait.

_____

_____

REVIEW QUESTIONS

1. What is the time period for prenatal development and postnatal development?

_____

_____

2. Why is capacitation necessary for fertilization?

_____

_____

3. Where does fertilization usually take place, and on what day of the menstrual cycle is it likely to occur?

_____

_____

4. What is the name of the single cell that is the result of fertilization? How many chromosomes does it have?

_____

5. How long does the pre-embryonic period last, and what developmental events occur during this time?

_____

_____

6. What are the three parts of a blastocyst?

_____

_____

_____

7. What hormone is secreted by the trophoblast cells, and what is its function?

_____

_____

_____

8. Name the primary germ layers, and list five derivatives from each one.

9. How long does the period of embryonic development last, and what takes place during this time?

_____

_____

10. What is the function of the (A) amnion, (B) chorion, (C) yolk sac, (D) allantois, (E) placenta?

A. _____

B. _____

C. _____

D. _____

E. _____

11. How long does the fetal period development last, and what two fundamental processes take place during this period?

_____

_____

12. What is the purpose of each of the following: (A) umbilical arteries, (B) umbilical vein, (C) ductus venosus, (D) foramen ovale, (E) ductus arteriosus?

A. _____

B. _____

C. _____

D. _____

E. _____

13. What is the normal length of time form fertilization until parturition?

_____

14. What hormone from the posterior pituitary stimulates uterine contractions during labor?

_____

15. List the three stages of labor and describe what take place in each stage.

_____

_____

_____

_____

16. Why does an infant's first breath need to be especially strong and forceful?

_____

17. What normally happens to each of the following after birth? (A) umbilical arteries, (B) umbilical vein, (C) ductus venosus, (D) foramen ovale, (E) ductus arteriosus?

A. _____

B. _____

C. _____

D. _____

E. _____

18. When is colostrum produced? What is the difference between colostrum and milk?

_____

_____

19. What is the role of the mother's hypothalamus in providing milk for a nursing infant?

_____

_____

20. What effects do estrogen and progesterone have on the structure of the mammary glands?

_____

_____

21. How does the posterior pituitary affect the mammary glands?

_____

22. Define six periods of life between birth and death.

_____

_____

_____

_____

_____

23. What is the difference between a chromosome and a gene?

_____

_____

24. What is the mechanism of gene function? How do genes work?

_____

_____

25. Distinguish between (A) dominant gene and recessive gene, (B) homozygous and heterozygous, (C) genotype and phenotype.

A. _____

B. _____

C. _____

26. What is a Punnett square, and how it is used?

_____

_____

27. How does sex-linked inheritance differ from autosomal inheritance?

_____

_____

28. What is a mutation?

_____

_____

VOCABULARY PRACTICE

Match the definitions on the left with the correct clinical term from the column on the right by placing the corresponding letter in the space before the definition. Not all terms will be used.

1. _____	Act of giving birth to an infant	A. Amnion
2. _____	Innermost fetal membrane	B. Eclampsia
3. _____	Preparations that reduce or inhibit uterine contractions	C. Embryo
		D. Eutocia
4. _____	Woman who has borne more than one child	E. Fetus
5. _____	An agent that causes physical defects in a developing embryo	F. Lochia
6. _____	Period during which organ systems develop	G. Multipara
7. _____	Synthetic oxytocin	H. Neonate
8. _____	Good, normal childbirth	I. Parturition
9. _____	Vaginal discharge during the first 2 weeks after childbirth	J. Pitocin
		K. Teratogen
10. _____	Infant during first month after birth	L. Tocolytics

11. Write the meaning of the following abbreviations.

A. _____ GYN   F. _____ FAS

B. _____ SIDS   G. _____ OB

C. _____ EDD   H. _____ CVS

D. _____ FHR   I. _____ TAB

E. _____ LMP   J. _____ NB

12. Spelling is important in scientific and medical applications because only one or two incorrect letters can change the meaning. Circle the correctly spelled word for each of the following pairs.

A. gestation   jestation
B. corion   chorion
C. senescence   senesance
D. zona pellucida   zona pelucida
E. clostrum   colostrums

13. Write the meaning of the underlined portion of each word on the line preceding the word.

A. _____ amniorrhea

B. _____ contraceptive

C. _____ pseudocyesis

D. _____ primigravida

E. _____ nullipara

F. _____ prenatal

G. _____ amniocentesis

H. _____ zygote

I. _____ dystocia

J. _____ senescence

14. Use your knowledge of word parts from all chapters to write definitions of the following words.

A. amniorrhea _____

B. contraceptive _____

C. pseudocyesis _____

D. primigravida _____

293

E. nullipara   _____

F. prenatal   _____

G. amniocentesis   _____

H. zygote   _____

I. dystocia   _____

J. senescence   _____

15. For each of the following words, underline the word part that corresponds to the underlined word or phrase in the definition.

A. cleavage	early <u>divisions</u> of the zygote into blastomeres
B. blastocyst	<u>hollow</u> ball of cells that results from cleavage
C. morphogenesis	developmental changes in <u>shape and form</u>
D. morula	ball of blastomeres that resembles a <u>mulberry</u>
E. nulliparous	bearing <u>no</u> children
F. oxytocin	hormone to stimulate <u>rapid</u> birth
G. parturition	the process of <u>giving birth</u>

16. There were complications in Clacy's pregnancy because of an abnormal implantation of the placenta in the lower portion of the uterus.

A. What is the clinical term for this condition?

    _____

B. During which prenatal period does the placenta develop?

    _____

C. Name three hormones produced by the placenta.

    _____

    _____

    _____

TESTING COMPREHENSION

Multiple choice: Select the best response.

1. Fertilization of an egg usually occurs in the (a) vagina, (b) cervix, (c) body of the uterus, (d) uterine tube.

2. Which of the following does *not* occur in the preembryonic period? (a) formation of the yolk sac, (b) cleavage, (c) formation of the ectoderm, (d) zygote implants in the uterine wall.

3. Capacitation occurs (a) during cleavage, (b) before fertilization, (c) during the pre-embryonic period, (d) while the ectoderm is forming.

4. The pre-embryonic period lasts for (a) 1 week; (b) 2 weeks; (c) 6 weeks; (d) 30 weeks.

5. The cells that are around the blastocele and contribute to the formation of the placenta make up the (a) blastocyst, (b) inner cell mass, (c) trophoblast, (d) morula.

6. Implantation in the endometrium *begins* about (a) 7 days after ovulation, (b) 7 hours after ovulation, (c) 7 days after the last menstrual period, (d) 14 days after ovulation.

7. Human chorionic gonadotropin (a) promotes cleavage, (b) maintains the corpus luteum, (c) contributes to the formation of the germ layers, (d) converts the corpus luteum into the corpus albicans.

8. Arrange the following events in the correct sequence: (1) formation of the inner cell mass, (2) cleavage, (3) appearance of lanugo hair, (4) formation of the primary germ layers, (5) heart starts beating. (a) 1, 2, 4, 3, 5; (b) 2, 1, 5, 3, 4; (c) 4, 1, 2, 5, 3; (d) 2, 1, 4, 5, 3.

9. How many primary germ layers are there? (a) one; (b) two; (c) three; (d) four.

10. Structures that develop from the ectoderm include the (a) lens of the eye and epidermis of the skin, (b) dermis of the skin and lining of the digestive tract, (c) cartilage and bone, (d) dermis of the skin and cartilage.

11. Which of the extraembryonic membranes contributes to the formation of the placenta? (a) amnion, (b) chorion, (c) yolk sac, (d) allantois.

12. The source of the primordial germ cells is the (a) amnion, (b) chorion, (c) yolk sac, (d) placenta.

13. Which of the following is *not* a function of the amniotic fluid? (a) maintains constant pressure and temperature around the embryo, (b) provides conditions for symmetrical development, (c) provides freedom of movement for development of muscles and bones, (d) provides nourishment for the developing embryo.

14. If a pregnant woman is 45 days past the beginning of her last menstrual period, the developing offspring is (a) in the cleavage stage of development, (b) in the pre-embryonic stage of development, (c) in the embryonic stage of development, (d) in the fetal stage of development.

15. Which of the following is *not* true about the placenta? (a) it forms from both embryonic and maternal tissue; (b) blood-filled lacunae in the endometrium surround chorionic villi; (c) maternal blood enters the chorionic villi to provide oxygen for the fetus; (d) it is expelled in the placental stage of labor.

16. Which of the following hormones is *not* secreted by the placenta? (a) prolactin, (b) estrogen, (c) progesterone, (d) human chorionic gonadotropin.

17. One day during class, Carmen felt her baby move within her uterus. This movement is called (a) caseosa, (b) quickening, (c) lanugo, (d) shifting.

18. The vessel between the umbilical vein and inferior vena cava is the (a) umbilical artery, (b) ductus venosus, (c) ductus arteriosus, (d) internal iliac artery.

19. The birth of an infant is called (a) gestation, (b) parturition, (c) labor, (d) lactation.

20. Which of the following occurs during the longest stage of labor? (a) the amniotic sac ruptures, (b) the baby passes through the birth canal, (c) the placenta is expelled, (d) the foramen ovale closes.

21. Which of the following hormones is most responsible for milk production when breast feeding an infant? (a) human chorionic gonadotropin, (b) estrogen, (c) prolactin, (d) oxytocin.

22. Which of the following does *not* refer to the neonatal period? (a) begins at the moment of birth, (b) foramen ovale normally closes, (c) temperature regulating mechanisms may not be fully developed, (d) baby learns to smile and laugh.

23. How may autosomes does a human normally have? (a) 22 pairs, (b) 46, (c) 1 pair, (d) 23.

24. If the mother has type AB blood and the father has type O blood, then (a) all sons will have type O blood, (b) daughters may be type A or type B, (c) half the sons will be type AB and half will be type O, (d) half the daughters will be type A and half will be type O.

25. Monosomy and trisomy result from (a) nondisjunction during meiosis, (b) genetic mutation during meiosis, (c) teratogens during meiosis, (d) segregation during meiosis.

A STEP BEYOND

Go a step beyond the ordinary and learn more about a topic that is related to this chapter but not discussed in detail in the textbook. Select one of the following topics, or one suggested by your instructor, and write a brief paper (250 words minimum), create a poster, or develop a short presentation (approximately 4 to 5 minutes) that focuses on your selection. Suggested topics for this chapter:

1. Fetal alcohol syndrome (FAS). What is it? What are its characteristics? How is the diagnosis made? What problems occur in children with FAS?
2. Teratogens. What are teratogens, and what are their features? What are some common teratogens? Select one the common teratogens and investigate its effects.
3. Tetralogy of Fallot. What is the tetralogy of Fallot? What are the four congenital heart defects involved? How do they affect the circulatory patterns of the infant? What are the signs and symptoms? How is it diagnosed and treated? What is the prognosis?
4. Down syndrome. What is Down syndrome, and how is it diagnosed? What is the chromosome basis? What are the signs and symptoms? How frequently does it occur?
5. Inherited blood disorders. Select one of the inherited blood disorders, such as hemophilia, thalassemia, or sickle cell anemia. Investigate the genetic basis of the disorder and how it is inherited. Learn about the signs and symptoms, diagnosis, and treatment.

FUN & GAMES

Word Scramble

Determine the word that fits each definition, and then write the word in the spaces across from the definition, one letter per space. The letters in the boxes form a scrambled word or words. Unscramble the letters to create a word that matches the final definition in each section.

1. Mitotic cell divisions after fertilization

2. Membrane that forms a sac around the embryo

3. Primary germ layer that forms the skin

4. Hormone that stimulates milk production

Letters to use for final word: _____.

Final definition: Process that weakens the membrane around the acrosome

_____

5. One of two or more alternative forms of genes at the same site on a chromosome

6. Visible expression of genes for a given trait

7. Solid ball of cells resulting from cleavage

8. Cluster of cells that becomes the embryo

9. Extraembryonic membrane that becomes part of the umbilical cord

Letters to use for final word: _____

Final definition: Surgical procedure used to obtain a sample of fluid from around the fetus

_____